Treatment Planning for the Developing Dentition

Quintessentials of Dental Practice – 26
Paediatric Dentistry/Orthodontics – 3

Treatment Planning for the Developing Dentition

By
Helen Rodd
Alyson Wray

Editor-in-Chief: Nairn H F Wilson
Editor Paediatric Dentistry/Orthodontics: Marie Thérèse Hosey

Quintessence Publishing Co. Ltd.

London, Berlin, Chicago, Paris, Milan, Barcelona, Istanbul,
São Paulo, Tokyo, New Delhi, Moscow, Prague, Warsaw

British Library Cataloguing-in Publication Data

Rodd, Helen
  Treatment planning for the developing dentition. - (Quintessentials of
  dental practice; 26)
  1. Pedodontics 2. Dental therapeutics - Planning
  I. Title II. Wray, Alison III. Wilson, Nairn H. F. IV. Hosey, Marie Therese
  617.6´45

  ISBN 1850970815

ISBN 1-85097-081-5

Foreword

Good treatment planning for the developing dentition gives the child patient life-long benefits. Indeed, getting things right in the management of developing dentitions may make a major contribution to many more patients enjoying the benefits of having teeth and oral health for life. Treatment planning for the developing dentition is therefore an onerous responsibility, with tremendous implications for patients, let alone oral healthcare systems. Furthermore, there is enormous professional fulfilment in seeing young patients mature dentally fit, subsequent to effective management in the developing dentition phase of their formative years.

Treatment Planning for the Developing Dentition, Volume 26 in the very successful *Quintessentials* series, gives excellent, new insight into the many, interlinked complexities of the management of the developing dentition. The need to adopt a forward-looking, holistic approach to developing dentition management is the thrust of this most helpful book. Needless to say, being a volume of the *Quintessentials* series, this addition to the dental literature is well produced, easy to read and attractively illustrated. In congratulating the authors on a job well done, I am pleased to recommend this *Quintessentials* volume to all those who care, and anticipate caring for patients with a developing dentition. I consider it a disappointing day if I do not learn something new about clinical dentistry. The day I read *Treatment Planning for the Developing Dentition* was a very good day, given all that I learnt about the complexity of the development of the dentition. Hopefully, you, like me, will find this book both informative and most worthwhile − a pleasure to read and a reliable text for future reference.

Nairn Wilson
Editor-in-Chief

Acknowledgements

We would like to express our thanks to a number of people who have helped us with this book. First, we are very grateful to Nairn Wilson (Editor-in-Chief) and Marie Thérèse Hosey (Editor) for their meticulous review of the text and constructive comments. Thanks are also due to our colleagues Iain Buchanan, Sarah North and Zoe Marshman for their valuable advice.

We would like to acknowledge the Medical Illustration Departments of Sheffield Teaching Hospitals NHS Trust and Glasgow Dental Hospital (Gail Drake, in particular) for the excellent clinical photography. A number of colleagues also provided some figures for inclusion in this book - Ian Ball (Figs 2-11, 2-12(b), 2-15(b), 2-16(a, b), 3-11(c), Iain Buchanan (Figs 1-6, 2-5(a, b), 2-13), Sally Craig (2-14(b), 4-7, 5-3(a, b), 5-16), Peter Robinson (5-19) and Melanie Stern (Figs 2-6, 6-3).

Dr Rodd would like to take the opportunity to thank her Sheffield orthodontic colleagues Melanie Stern, Fiona Dyer, Philip Benson and Derrick Willmot for their constant readiness to give advice and support for any patient at any time. Thanks are also extended to the Derbyshire Craft Centre Cafe for the free coffees during proof-reading sessions and to James Marson for his support in every endeavour.

Dr Wray would like to thank particularly Iain Buchanan for his willingness to review Chapter 2 and for providing constructive advice. Thanks also to Fiona Gilchrist and to Cameron and Blythe Wray for help with clinical photographs. Finally, thanks to David Wray for making the time available to allow completion of this manuscript.

Preface

Treatment planning is the foundation of good clinical practice. But how much time and thought is actually put into a treatment plan? For some practitioners, the process may be intuitive, while others may spend considerable time weighing up the pros and cons of alternative plans according to each patient's particular needs and circumstances. Whatever the approach, we hope this book will help to outline some principles of good treatment planning for the young patient. Treatment planning for children involves greater responsibility than for most patients. As early dental experiences may shape future behaviour and attitudes, the aim is to ensure that the child has a pleasant and positive introduction to dentistry. Good dental care in childhood helps attain a healthy, functional and aesthetic adult dentition. Conversely, ill-made decisions at an early age may lead to a compromised dentition in later life.

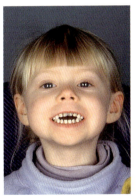 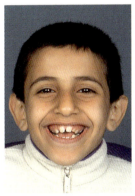 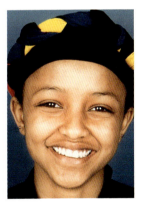

Dental care of children requires individual treatment planning.

A good treatment plan should be:

- Realistic – don't expect too much from young patients.
- Personalised – every child has different social, medical and dental needs; one treatment plan definitely doesn't fit all.

- Holistic – a treatment plan is not just a sequence of procedures, but something that, in children, includes behaviour-shaping, prevention and interceptive orthodontics.
- Flexible – circumstances and dental status change, therefore a treatment plan should not be too rigid.
- Progressive – it is essential to introduce children gradually to the more demanding aspects of their treatment plan, rather than diving in, for example, with a dental block on the first visit.
- Forward-thinking – it is important to consider the longer-term picture, keeping options open or carrying out interventions that may avoid, or at least reduce, the complexity of future treatment.

Spending time to develop a treatment plan is not only beneficial for the young patient and their parents, but it also helps the operator by:

- reducing stress levels
- optimising time management
- increasing job satisfaction.

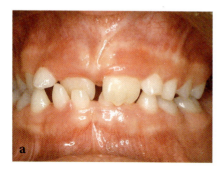
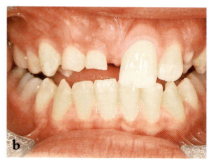
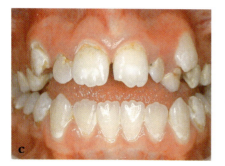

A spectrum of treatment planning challenges: (a) eight-year-old with anterior cross-bite and severe hypodontia (b) 10-year-old with clinically absent upper right permanent central and lateral incisors (c) 13-year-old with rampant caries and orthodontic crowding.

Skilled treatment planners are much less likely to run into difficulties with patients refusing to cooperate or agitated parents who claim not to know what is going on. Certainly, litigation problems are substantially reduced if one can demonstrate a comprehensive treatment plan for each patient that has been discussed and agreed with all concerned. As we are now increasingly working with professionals complementary to dentistry, it is mandatory that we provide these colleagues with a clearly itemised programme of treatment for young patients. This book does not set out to dictate rigid treatment plans for every clinical scenario, but rather aims to explain the basic principles behind good decision-making. On reading this book we would hope that the reader would have an understanding of the following:

- the importance of the child's first visit to gain all information necessary to form a comprehensive treatment plan
- the importance of interceptive orthodontic treatment planning
- the preventive phase of a treatment plan
- the restorative phase of a treatment plan
- how to manage the emergency presentation
- recall strategies for the young patient.

Helen Rodd & Alyson Wray

Contents

Chapter 1
The First Visit

Aim

In this chapter the importance of introducing a young child to dentistry is emphasised and a strategy for structuring dental treatment is outlined.

Objectives

After reading this chapter the dentist should be able to:

- understand the importance of the child's early impressions
- plan first visits according to the age of the child
- appreciate the need for a thorough history and clinical examination
- undertake caries risk assessment
- understand the need to initiate a hierarchical treatment plan.

Introduction

Children are the adult dental patients of the future, and good groundwork in the early years of dental monitoring and treatment planning will pay dividends in both the short and long term (Fig 1-1). Furthermore, children are infinitely variable in their behaviour, their development and in their dental needs, and therefore one of the key aims of this book is to establish the importance of individualising treatment planning and dental care.

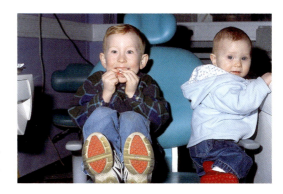

Fig 1-1 Two pre-school children exploring the dental environment.

1

There are many reasons why appropriate treatment planning is important – for example, the avoidance of unnecessary treatment such as repeat general anaesthetics or endodontic treatment on a tooth with an unrestorable crown, the facilitation of future interventions, such as retaining roots to maintain alveolar bone, and reduction in stress for operators and patients. It is particularly important with young patients to set easily achievable targets for each visit and for the overall treatment plan. The overall aims of a course of treatment may be very different from those for an adult patient.

First Visit – First Impressions

We are all aware that first impressions can be lasting ones. It is very important that any child's introduction to dentistry leaves as favourable an impression as possible. This is one of the many reasons why it is so helpful if children begin attending when they have no immediate treatment need. A child who first attends in pain and who may require operative treatment at that visit will have a very different first impression from one who attends symptom-free and only requires a dental examination. For an overview of the approach for a child presenting in pain see Chapter 5.

It is usually beneficial to give children a morning appointment. Although parents may be resistant to this, preferring appointments after school, many young children are tired and hungry at this time of day, and their behaviour is affected accordingly. Seeing young children in the morning, when you are both relatively fresh, is usually more productive.

Wherever possible the practice environment should be child-friendly. Bright decorations, good lighting, simple toys or games in the waiting area go a long way to making a positive first impression. All appointments run late from time to time, but ideally children, in particular anxious ones, should not be kept waiting. If waiting is unavoidable, toys, storybooks and appropriate videos will help to make the wait more pleasant (Fig 1-2).

Dental practices are very busy places, and it is commonplace for the dentist to stay in the surgery for most of the session and have the dental nurse go to the waiting room to escort the patients to the surgery. This is usually acceptable for adult patients, and those who are very familiar with, and relaxed in, the dental environment. For new, young patients it is much less intimidating if the dentist greets the child in the waiting room, with an accompanying adult close at hand, and then escorts the child into the surgery. Remember that eye contact is very important, in particular at a first meeting. It may

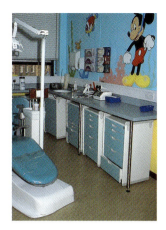
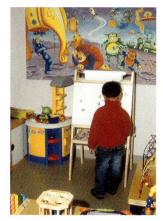
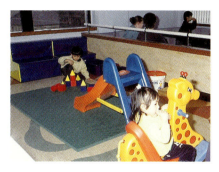

Fig 1-2
Child-friendly
surgery and
waiting areas.

be necessary to bend down, or even kneel, to make good eye contact with a small child. Communication involves words (verbal), tone and actions (non-verbal). With children, the verbal component is the least important.

Parent in or out of the Surgery: the Treatment Triangle

Whether or not to have parents in the dental surgery during treatment of their child is an issue most dentists feel quite strongly about. Some advocate always having parents present, others would say never. In reality, it is probably inappropriate to have a hard and fast rule. It is well documented that separation anxiety begins to develop in children around the age of eight or nine months, usually peaks around two to three years of age and for most has dwindled again by the age of five. It would seem reasonable, therefore, to have children accompanied by their parent or carer until the age of three or four, and to make individual decisions about accompaniment from then

3

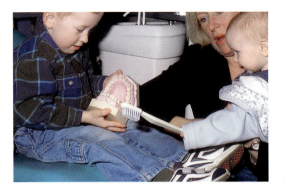

Fig 1-3 Parental presence is important to reassure very young children in an unfamiliar environment.

on (Fig 1-3). A self–confident four-year-old who knows the dentist well will happily sit for a check-up on his or her own. An anxious five-year-old, new to the practice, who needs a first local anaesthetic should, however, have a parent present, provided that the parent has a positive effect on the child's behaviour.

It is helpful to establish with the parent that his or her role is to provide support for the child, not to become a communication barrier between the dentist and the patient. An outline of the pros and cons of having parents in the surgery is given in Table 1-1. More detail is given in another volume in this series, *Child Taming* (see recommended reading).

The Child is Part of the Family

Before any treatment plan can be drafted, the process of information-gathering must be completed. This can begin even before the first visit, as many children will be part of families already attending the practice. Thus knowledge of the family's attitude towards dentistry and dental treatment, together with the family history of dental needs, provides a useful base for treatment planning.

Ideally young children should be regular dental attenders as part of family visits from the time of tooth eruption. In reality many children do not attend for dental care until the age of three or four, or until they are experiencing symptoms. Later in this chapter some examples of treatment plans for different age groups are given by way of suggestions for the possible structuring of a series of appointments.

Table 1-1 **An outline of the pros and cons of having parents in the surgery**

Pro	Con
• Increases parent/ dentist communication • Parent witnesses first hand the child's behaviour • Time saved answering questions • Children aged three and under benefit psychologically from the parents' presence	• Parent often repeats orders to the annoyance of both the dentist and the child • The parent interjects in conversation, becoming a barrier to good communication between the dentist and the child • The dentist is unable to use stern voice intonation, in case the parent is offended • The child divides his attention between the parent and the dentist • The dentist divides his attention between the child and the parent • Parental anxiety may have a negative effect on child's behaviour

Information Gathering

There are varying opinions regarding the degree of formality appropriate between the dentist and the patient: where children are concerned, it is usually helpful to be informal and to proceed on first-name terms. There are no hard and fast rules, however, and there is scope for individual preferences. Once introductions are complete and the child has been escorted into the surgery, the information-gathering process can begin. It is all too easy to assume that an accompanying adult is the child's parent but, in fact, members of the extended family, child-minders, even neighbours often bring children to the dentist. It is therefore important to always ask the specific question 'Are you the mother/father?' to preclude misunderstandings. Some children will immediately climb up into the dental chair, but others are hesitant and need more time to become confident. It is helpful to establish a rapport around a subject of relevance and interest to each individual child. A few moments discussing non-dental topics, such as siblings, school or nursery, favourite toys, TV programmes, special holidays or birthdays can provide a wealth of information for both immediate and future use. Making a brief note of special interests on the record card comes in handy at the six-month recall.

Most children have inquisitive minds and lively imaginations. They benefit from being given a clear understanding of what is about to happen and from being given the opportunity to ask questions. Giving small children the dental mirror to hold, allowing them to look at their own teeth and 'counting' the teeth with them are all helpful strategies. Giving children with an 'internal locus of control' lots of details about their forthcoming treatment helps them to feel in control: they believe they can control what happens to them and are more likely to take preventive actions and to be responsible for their own care.

Children with an 'external locus of control' believe what happens to them is by chance or luck and can only be influenced by someone other than themselves, for example the dentist. This type of child tends to respond best to being given only an outline of their treatment: giving too much detail only makes them feel more anxious. It is very helpful to quickly identify which group any individual young patient might belong to.

At the first visit for a very young child, in particular an anxious child, the optimum time to stop may come after only a few minutes. Letting the patient leave the surgery with a sense of achievement is a powerful incentive to come back. For some children, just sitting in the dental chair and allowing an examination is a milestone.

The History

An appropriate treatment plan depends on good history-taking. This is a multistage process, which is often done so skilfully by an experienced practitioner that the different stages are seamless. Any presenting complaint should be established at the outset, as this is often the reason for attendance, and it is important that this is not overlooked. It is also very helpful to establish why children think they are in the surgery, as they may have a very different perspective from everyone else.

The past dental history for a child patient maybe very short, but it can still provide useful information. Of particular importance is the history of compliance with any operative techniques and the administration of local anaesthetic. If there have been any negative past experiences, it is very important to take note of these: it is often much easier to give a child the first local anaesthetic than it is to give a second when there has been an uncomfortable first experience. Any history of dental trauma may be important, as is any previous exposure to general anaesthesia for dental extractions.

The medical history is often very straightforward: the majority of children have had no significant illnesses, nor are they on any medication. A small portion of children will, however, have significant heart or chest conditions, allergies, behaviour problems, attention deficit hyperactivity disorder (ADHD) or a variety of other conditions that could have an impact on either their ability to cope with dental treatment or on the appropriateness of elements of a treatment plan.

Finally the social history, once again, is often straightforward, but increasing numbers of children do not live with two parents, and many do not live with either parent – all the more reason to establish who is accompanying the child. Only parents or legal guardians can give consent on behalf of a child for treatment, so it must be clear who these individuals are. The legal framework relating to consent for treatment varies in different parts of the UK, but it is every practitioner's responsibility to understand the relevant legislation.

The Clinical Picture

During the course of the examination a wide range of clinical information can be gathered. A note should be made of the child's attitude towards the examination process and the prospect of treatment. Many children are quite happy to sit in the chair and 'have their teeth counted' but shrink back in fear at the suggestion of a filling.

A brief extraoral examination should always be undertaken, noting any asymmetry, obvious malocclusion, perioral infection, bumps and bruises, secondary herpes infection (cold sores), head lice and so on. For the majority of children there will be little to note extraorally, but it is important not to overlook any obvious abnormalities in the haste to get inside the mouth.

Very young or frightened children are best examined on a parent's knee. If the child is less than three years old, the best technique is often to have the child facing the parent on their knee. The dentist sits directly facing the parent, with their knees almost touching. The child is then gently laid back-

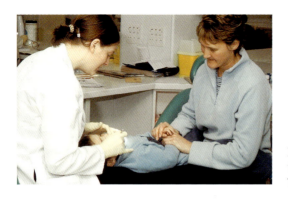

Fig 1-4 Recommended position for examination of a very young child.

wards onto the dentist's knee, but can still clearly see the parent, who can help with reassurance and physical contact. An older child with behavioural problems can also be examined on the parent's knee, or it may be necessary to postpone the first detailed examination for a future visit, unless symptoms dictate that early intervention is required (Fig 1-4).

The intraoral examination should include examination of the soft tissues before examination of the occlusion and then the teeth. Children are susceptible to viral infections of the oral soft tissues, such as primary herpes and herpangina. They may also be prone to recurrent aphthous ulceration, which occurs on the non-keratinised mucosa (Fig 1-5a–c).

A note should be made of any obvious occlusal abnormalities, such as an anterior open bite, cross-bite, marked crowding or spacing, atypical incisor relationship and the presence of a tongue tie (Fig 1-6a,b). More details on the assessment of the developing occlusion can be found in the next chapter.

The Dentition
Only once the history-taking and examination process have been completed should the dentition be scrutinised. An overall assessment of tooth quality can be made quickly. Caries most commonly determines tooth quality in the young patient. On occasions other factors, such as erosion, enamel hypomineralisation and hypoplasia and hereditary defects such as amelogenesis imperfecta, will have a profound influence on tooth quality. It is especially important to record a detailed dental charting in children, as their dentition changes dramatically over time, and delayed eruption or congenital absence of teeth may otherwise be missed (Fig 1-7a–d).

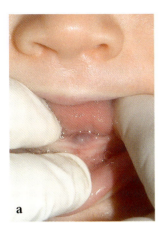

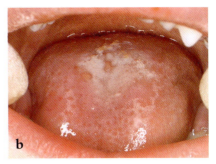

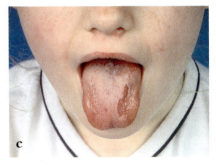

Fig 1-5 (a) Eruption cyst in a seven-month-old baby. (b) Primary herpes infection showing marked ulceration on the dorsum of the tongue. (c) The classic appearance of geographic tongue.

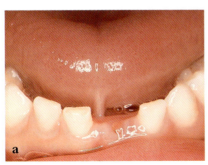

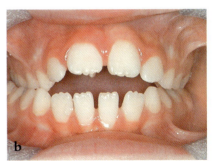

Fig 1-6 (a) Tongue tie. (b) Anterior open bite.

The following information should be recorded during the course of the intra-oral examination:

- erupted teeth
- incisor relationship
- carious teeth and surfaces

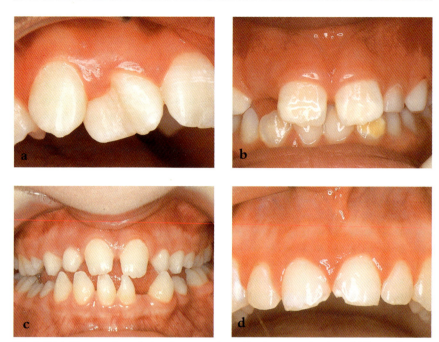

Fig 1-7 (a) Abnormal tooth development: lateral incisor germination. (b) Enamel opacities: hypomineralisation. (c) Congenitally missing teeth. (d) Classic appearance of thin, chipped incisal edges linked to palatal erosion.

- areas of decalcification
- restored teeth and surfaces, including the restorative material
- fissure-sealed teeth
- enamel defects, including opacities and hypoplasia
- palpable teeth (particularly permanent maxillary canines)
- any swelling/sinus/colour change noted in association with caries, heavily restored or traumatised teeth
- any mobile teeth
- any signs of erosion or abnormal attrition, such as thin or chipped edges
- oral hygiene status.

The assumption can usually be made that primary teeth absent before their expected age of exfoliation have been extracted as a consequence of caries. It is helpful to know whether these teeth were removed under general anaesthesia and, if so, at what age. The implications of these clinical findings are considered in more detail in Table 1-2.

Table 1-2 **Implications of some common clinical findings**

Clinical Finding	Relevance
• Erupted teeth	Appropriate for age/stage of development? Are others unerupted/ absent or extracted?
• Incisor relationship	Changes over developmental stages –may give early indication of developing malocclusion
• Carious teeth and surfaces	Key indicator of caries risk
• Areas of decalcification	Indicator of cariogenic diet and poor oral hygiene
• Restored teeth and surfaces and used restorative material(s)	Indicative of past caries activity and previous compliance with treatment
• Fissure sealed teeth	Indicative of some previous compliance with treatment
• Hypomineralised and hypoplastic teeth	Caries risk factor – may be aesthetic concern
• Palpable teeth	Indicative of imminent eruption – useful for locating tooth position
• Swelling/sinus/colour change noted in association with caries or traumatised teeth	Indicative of loss of vitality and infection
• Mobile teeth	Check whether mobility is physio- logical (tooth is near exfoliation) or pathological (indicative of infection or bone loss)
• Evidence of erosion or excessive attrition	Indicative of high frequency of intake of carbonated drinks or other erosive foodstuffs. Attrition age four to five years in primary dentition is usually not a cause of concern
• Oral hygiene status	Indicative of caries risk, attitude to dental treatment and manual dexterity

Radiographic Assessment?

Once the clinical picture is complete an informed decision can be made about the need for a radiographic examination (Fig 1-8). Radiographs are most frequently indicated for caries assessment, and in such cases bitewing radiographs are the preferred view. Lateral oblique views can, however, be considered for children who cannot tolerate an intraoral film, although the value of this view is variable. Where the contact areas are not closed – for example, because the second primary molars have only recently erupted, primary molar extractions have been undertaken or there is a spaced dentition - a radiographic investigation for caries may not be indicated at all.

Panoramic radiographs are sometimes indicated to assess dental development or to check for suspected pathology. Other views are required from time to

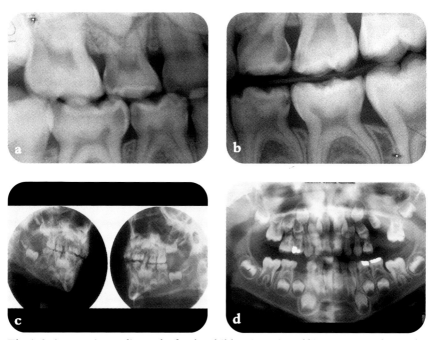

Fig 1-8 Appropriate radiographs for the child patient. (a and b) Bitewing radiographs are the view of choice for detecting caries. (c) In skilled hands, lateral oblique views are useful for assessing dental development, or where co-operation for intra-oral views is poor. (d) Panoramic views are also useful for assessing dental development or where pathology is suspected in a number of different areas.

time, including periapical views for caries assessment in permanent anterior teeth, or for endodontic treatment and for the diagnosis and monitoring of traumatic injuries. Occasionally two views are required to locate unerupted teeth, supernumeraries or root fractures. A guide to the appropriate use of radiographs in children, for both new and recall patients, is given in Table 1-3.

Caries Risk Assessment

There are two main purposes to this information-gathering process. The first is to establish the caries risk category of the patient. The second is to use the

Table 1-3 **A guide to the appropriate use of radiographs in children**

	Primary Dentition	**Mixed Dentition**	**Permanent Dentition**
New patient	Bitewing or lateral oblique views (if bitewings not tolerated)	Bitewings, together with panoramic, occlusal and periapical views, if indicated clinically	Bitewings, together with panoramic, occlusal and periapical views, if indicated clinically
Recall patient			
High caries risk	Bitewings 6- to 12-monthly	Bitewings 6- to12-monthly	Bitewings 12-monthly
Low caries risk	Bitewings 12- to 24-monthly	Bitewings 12- to 24-monthly	Bitewings 24- to 36-monthly
Growth and development	Not usually indicated. Panoramic view where specific problem suspected	Panoramic view to monitor developing occlusion, or to plan extractions of permanent teeth	Panoramic view to monitor development/ position of third permanent molars

risk assessment to develop an individualised treatment plan. Risk assessment for dental caries is based on three key factors:

- clinical findings
- dental development
- other findings.

A list of the relevant factors in each of these categories is given in Table 1-4. It is helpful to note on the patient's record card their risk category - this may change with time. In fact, the aim should be to get all patients into the low-risk category and to keep them there.

Why is this an important process? The risk category helps to determine the most appropriate treatment plan. For example, when faced with a five-year-old with extensive caries in all four first primary molars and more moderate cavities in the second primary molars, with little home support

Table 1-4 **Caries risk assessment factors**

Clinical	Social and Behavioural	Developmental
• Decalcification	• Multiple sugar intakes	• Appropriate for age?
• Considerable plaque	• Irregular attendance	• Symmetrical lesions
• Extractions due to caries	• Mother has high caries rate	• Teeth recently erupted? For example, Es at two-and-a-half years, 6s at six to seven years and 7s at 12 years: teeth are at increased caries risk in the first year post-eruption
• Hypomineralised or hypoplastic teeth	• No fluoride / irregular brushing	
• Primary dentition crowding	• Prolonged breast-feeding after tooth eruption	
• Salivary factors	• Bottle-feeding during the night	

for tooth-brushing and diet modification (very definitely high risk), a decision to restore strategic teeth (second primary molars) could be justified, along with intensive prevention, frequent recalls and regular radiographic examination. In contrast, if an eight-year-old patient presents with some caries in the first primary molars only it would be appropriate to consider this individual as moderate risk and to adopt a 'less aggressive' preventive, radiographic and recall strategy.

Treatment Planning

The reasons it is important to have a detailed treatment plan for the dental care of a child are as follows:

- For a clear understanding of the treatment proposed, thereby facilitating informed consent
- To gauge how much time will be involved in completing treatment, both for the dentist, and for the parent and patient to plan time off work and school and, where appropriate, to arrange child care for siblings
- To facilitate a hierarchy of treatment - in particular, for young, anxious patients - to allow them to gradually adapt to more demanding treatments
- To avoid unnecessary treatment, such as restoring teeth that would be better extracted, or minimising the risk of repeated dental general anaesthesia
- For legal reasons.

Balancing all the variables gathered during the history and examination process, and using this information to create a customised treatment plan, requires a high level of experience and skill. Care must be taken to consider the parent's motivation, the child's likely compliance and the access to dental services, such as general anaesthesia and sedation. The complexity of all these interactions ensures that no two treatment plans are identical. In preference to outlining a long list of treatment options, a few common scenarios are given below. These cover some of the most frequently occurring situations.

An important feature of a successful treatment plan in Paediatric Dentistry is the incorporation of three key components into each visit, namely: prevention, acclimatisation and operative techniques. Not only should these three components be present at each visit, but they also need to be introduced in a hierarchical manner. For example, in order to complete a small two-surface restoration in an anxious six-year-old, a large number of 'mini'-

procedures have to be explained and experienced before the procedure can be completed. For example:
- overhead light on, safety glasses on, chair reclined
- patient happy to keep mouth wide open
- accepting cotton rolls/dry guards
- accepting the saliva ejector
- topical anaeasthetic
- local anaesthetic
- three-in-one syringe
- aspirator
- handpieces: high and slow speed
- hand instrumentation
- matrix band
- strange-tasting dental materials
- curing light
- final adjustments and finishing.

Clearly, from the child's perspective the above is far too much to introduce all at one visit. It is not surprising that many children only get to stage four or five on this list before clamping their teeth together and refusing to cooperate further. The fact that they are likely to be labelled 'uncooperative' from then on is unfair.

A much higher likelihood of success may be achieved with the following approach:

Visit 1
Carry out examination in the chair, give dietary advice, toothbrushing instruction, demonstration of the three-in-one syringe and saliva ejector.

Visit 2
Reinforce oral hygiene and dietary advice (Fig 1-9), demonstrate slow-speed handpiece and complete prophylaxis, introduce the patient to the curing light.

Visit 3
Apply fissure sealants using three-in-one syringe, aspirator, slow-speed handpiece and curing light. Introduce topical anaesthetic, give fluoride mouthwash.

Visit 4
Apply topical anaesthetic, infiltrate local anaesthetic, complete restoration

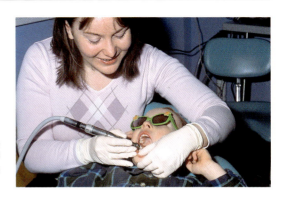

Fig 1-9 Completion of visit 2, as outlined above, with the patient and the dentist both pleased with the outcome.

with slow-speed or high-speed handpiece as appropriate, restore with light-cured compomer.

Although this is time-consuming, a structured hierarchical approach will save significant time in the longer term and produce a relaxed and cooperative patient for the future.

Sample Treatment Plans

Scenario 1

This is the first dental visit for a three-year-old girl. Her family are regular attenders. She is shy but not anxious and cooperates for a clinical examination, which reveals caries (cavitation) on all four first primary molars and some plaque deposits on the buccal surfaces of the molars. She is unable to cooperate for bitewing radiographs, but can manage lateral obliques. The caries in the first primary molars has not reached the pulp.

Caries risk: *Moderate*

Visit	Acclimatisation	Prevention	Operative
Visit 1	Examination, show teeth in mirror	Toothbrushing demonstration	Show handpiece: polish finger nails

Visit 2	Show handpiece, three-in-one syringe, curing light	Check tooth-brushing technique	Full mouth prophylaxis, apply fluoride varnish to lesions of caries
Visit 3	Show hand instruments, excavators and plastic instruments. Demonstrate aspirator	Explain diet diary to patient and parent	Open one cavity up with slow speed and remove caries with excavators. Restore with compomer. Explain that not all caries is removed
Visit 4	Consider introduction of topical and local anaesthetic if restorations will require it	Go over diet diary and offer constructive comments and changes	As above; if managing well consider doing two restorations
Visit 5	Reassess progress and cooperation: if local anaesthetic is possible then definitive restorations can be placed	Introduce fluoride supplements. Reinforce diet advice	As above; if local anaesthetic can be used at this stage, consider removal of all caries and placement of preformed crowns

Recall strategy: in view of the child's age and caries risk, recall every three to six months until risk category changes. Consider repeat bitewings in six to 12 months

Scenario 2

A nine-year-old boy presents for the first time with occasional pain in a lower left first permanent molar. His only previous experience of dental treatment is extractions under general anaesthetic. He is anxious, will allow an examination but is nervous of hand instruments and dislikes the chair being reclined. Clinical examination reveals caries in all four first permanent molars. The upper molars are restorable. Primary molars have previously been removed under general anaesthetic. A panoramic radiograph reveals the possibility of significant crowding. All the remaining permanent teeth are developing. The patient's oral hygiene is poor.

Caries risk: *High*

Visit	Acclimatisation	Prevention	Operative
Visit 1	Examination, show teeth in mirror, show teeth on radiograph and explain options. Consider sedation or general anaesthetic for extraction of first permanent molars	Toothbrushing demonstration, disclosing plaque, give fluoride mouth rinse	Show handpiece; full mouth prophylaxis; place sedative dressing in symptomatic tooth
Visit 2	Discuss options for extractions - pros and cons. Refer for general anaesthetic for removal of all first permanent molars	Check tooth-brushing technique, review plaque control; explain and issue diet diary	Fissure seal any cingulum pits
Visit 3	Review following general anaesthetic to re-establish contact	Go over diet diary and offer constructive comments and changes	Full mouth prophylaxis, fluoride varnish application

Recall strategy: in view of the boy's age and caries risk, recall in three months to review oral hygiene and diet diary. Monitor for signs of erosion. Remotivate. Maintain on frequent recalls until risk category reduces. Fissure seal premolars and second permanent molars on eruption

Scenario 3

A seven-year-old girl presents for annual recall. She has previously required three restorations in her primary molars, which she cooperated for with difficulty. The restorations have been replaced twice and are less than ideal. At this visit she has early caries in her first permanent molars, which erupted nine months ago. Her mother insists she hardly ever has sweets. Bitewing radiographs show the caries in the permanent teeth is into dentine, and the primary tooth restorations are deficient.

Caries risk: *High*

Visit	Acclimatisation	Prevention	Operative
Visit 1	Examination, show teeth in mirror	Toothbrushing demonstration; prescribe fluoride rinse	Show handpiece, full mouth prophylaxis
Visit 2	Introduce topical anaesthetic: explain that local anaesthetic will allow fillings to be completed painlessly	Check toothbrushing technique; explain diet diary to patient and parent	Remove the old restorations, hand-excavate as far as possible; dress temporarily
Visit 3	Demonstrate numbness from topical anaesthetic; demonstrate aspirator. Re-assess cooperation	Apply fluoride varnish to areas of decalcification; go over diet diary and make constructive comments and changes	Re-apply topical and administer local anaesthetic; remove dressing and caries from primary tooth; remove caries from permanent tooth in same quadrant; restore with compomer/composite and fissure seal

| **Visit 4** | Reassess progress and cooperation; consider inhalation sedation | Monitor and reinforce dietary changes | As above; complete upper quadrants first if possible |

Recall strategy: in view of age and caries risk, recall every three to six months until risk category changes. Apply fluoride varnish, monitor diet. Consider bitewings in six months

Recommended Reading

Chadwick B, Hosey MT. Child Taming: Managing Children in General Dental Practice. London: Quintessence Publishing, 2003.

Espelid I, Mejàre I, Weerheijm K. European Association of Paediatric Dentistry (EAPD) guidelines for the use of radiographs in children. European Journal of Paediatric Dentistry 2003;4:40-48.

Guthrie A. Separation anxiety: an overview. Pediatric Dentistry 1997;19:486-490.

Pitts NB, Kidd EAM. The prescription and timing of bitewing radiography in the diagnosis and management of dental caries: contemporary recommendations. British Dental Journal 1992;172:225-227.

Powell LV. Caries risk assessment: relevance to the practitioner. ASDC Journal of Dentistry for Children 1998;129:349-353.

Chapter 2

Interceptive Orthodontic Treatment

Aim

This chapter aims to establish the importance of good interceptive orthodontics for young dental patients.

Objectives

After reading this chapter the dentist should be able to:
- understand the importance of monitoring the developing dentition
- utilise a simple screening tool for the early identification of occlusal problems
- identify specific circumstances in which intervention may be beneficial
- have a clear understanding of which patients require referral and when this should occur.

Introduction

It is generally agreed that all children, from about six years of age, should be screened for the presence of a developing malocclusion when attending for a routine examination. Whilst the majority of orthodontic treatment is carried out in the late mixed or early permanent dentition, some conditions lend themselves to earlier treatment. A useful definition of interceptive orthodontics is: 'Any treatment designed to eliminate, or reduce the severity of a developing malocclusion'. The benefits of this interceptive treatment cannot be stressed enough. For example, early diagnosis and appropriate intervention may avoid the need for a much more prolonged course of treatment at a later stage (Fig 2-1a–c).

Table 2-1 outlines a number of possible problems to watch out for in the primary, mixed and early permanent dentition. The appropriate interceptive action for each of these conditions will be discussed in the subsequent sections.

The Developing 'Normal' Dentition

Malocclusion in the primary dentition is relatively rare. It is usually caused by

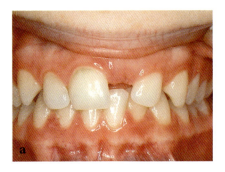

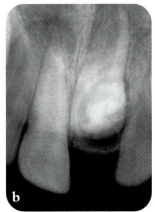

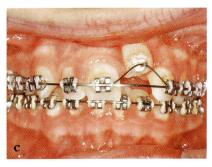

Fig 2-1 (a-c) The extensive amount of fixed orthodontic treatment necessary for a 13-year-old, simply because the space for the unerupted upper central incisor had not been maintained before tooth exposure.

environmental factors, such as digit-sucking habits and trauma. By the end of the primary dentition the anterior teeth are usually slightly spaced and often in an edge-to-edge relationship (Fig 2-2). If the primary teeth are 'well aligned' – that is, they have no spacing at the end of the primary dentition - then there is a very strong probability (>95%) that the permanent dentition will be crowded.

By definition, the mixed dentition is the developmental stage most conducive to interceptive orthodontics: it extends from the eruption of either the first permanent molars or the lower central incisors at around six to seven years of age, to the eruption of the second permanent molars and second pre-

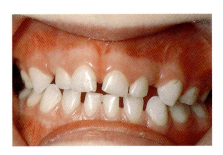

Fig 2-2 Normal spacing towards the end of the primary dentition.

Table 2-1 **An outline of possible problems to watch out for in the primary, early and late mixed dentition**

Primary Dentition	Early Mixed Dentition (six to nine years)	Late Mixed Dentition (10–12 years)
Not usually necessary to do anything – but watch out for things that may present as a problem later	*A critical time for appropriate monitoring and interceptive treatment*	*Should have already picked up all the problems listed for the early mixed dentition*
• lack of spacing indicates probable increased crowding in the permanent dentition	• delayed eruption especially upper incisors	• ectopic maxillary canines
• supernumerary teeth: 35–50% of cases will also have a permanent supernumerary	• deflected eruption due to retained primary tooth	• severe skeletal discrepancies
	• increased overjet	• traumatised anterior teeth of very poor prognosis
• congenitally missing teeth: hypodontia may be more severe in permanent dentition region	• crossbites especially if causing mandibular displacements, or if associated with localised gingival recession in the lower incisor	• crowding
• anterior open bite, may persist in permanent dentition	• deep overbite if causing trauma	
• crossbites may persist in permanent dentition	• anterior open bite: associated with digit-sucking?	
	• first permanent molars of poor prognosis	
	• infraoccluded teeth	
	• double teeth or teeth with abnormal morphology	
	• space loss, likely to occur following premature loss of second primary molars	
	• supernumerary teeth/congenitally missing teeth	

molars at around 11–12 years of age. The permanent teeth tend to erupt in two distinct phases: the incisors and first permanent molars from the age of six to eight-and-a-half, and the premolars, canines and second permanent molars from 10–12 years of age. There is an interim period of approximately two years when little changes, except for growth and an increase in the inter-canine width in both the upper and lower arches. A simple reminder of the eruption times for primary and permanent teeth is set out in Table 2-2. There is a reasonably wide inter-individual variation (± 6–12 months) in eruption times, particularly for different ethnic groups.

Screening for Problems

Numerous orthodontic assessment methods are described in the dental literature, but many are complex and designed for orthodontic treatment planning rather than as a practical screening tool. A simple screening tool is MOCDOO.

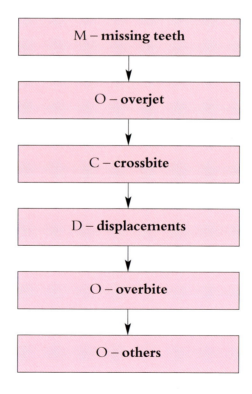

Table 2-2 **Eruption dates for primary and permanent teeth**

Dentition/Tooth	Eruption Time	Root Completed
Primary dentition		
Incisors		
Upper	7-9 months	18 months
Lower	6-8 months	18 months
First primary molars		
Upper	14-16 months	$2^{1/2}$ years
Lower	12-14 months	$2^{1/4}$ years
Primary canines		
Upper	18 months	$3^{1/4}$ years
Lower	16 months	$3^{1/4}$ years
Second primary molars		
Upper	2 years	3 years
Lower	20 months	3 years
Permanent dentition		
First permanent molars		
Upper	6-7 years	9-10 years
Lower	6-7 years	9-10 years
Central incisors		
Upper	7-8 years	10 years
Lower	6-7 year	9 years
Lateral incisors		
Upper	8-9 years	11 years
Lower	7-8 years	10 years
First premolars		
Upper	10-11 years	12-13 years
Lower	10-12 years	12-13 years
Second premolars		
Upper	10-12 years	12-14 years
Lower	11-12 years	13-14 years
Permanent canines		
Upper	11-12 years	13-15 years
Lower	9-10 years	12-14 years
Second permanent molars		
Upper	12-13 years	14-16 years
Lower	11-13 years	14-15 years
Third permanent molars		
Upper	17-21 years	18-25 years
Lower	17-21 years	18-25 years

This system is quick and easy to use, and will pick up most developing mal-occlusions if utilised regularly. We will now look at each particular category and briefly discuss appropriate interceptive treatment.

M – Missing Teeth

Teeth may be missing for a variety of reasons. They could be present but unerupted, or ectopically positioned. Alternatively, they could be congenitally absent. Don't discount the possibility that a tooth might be missing because it has been extracted and the parent has forgotten, or the child was brought for the extraction by the other parent.

Unerupted Teeth

The tooth which most frequently fails to erupt is the upper central incisor. The eruption of this tooth is often delayed by the presence of a supernumerary tooth, a retained primary tooth or occasionally by the presence of crown or root dilaceration following trauma. A useful rule of thumb is that paired teeth - for example, the upper central incisors - should erupt within six months of each other. If the eruption of the contralateral tooth is delayed more than this, further investigation is warranted (Fig 2-3a-e). A simplistic approach to the management of this problem may be as follows:

- Take a good history, including details of any previous trauma to the primary dentition, previous extractions or family history of missing teeth
- Palpate for the unerupted tooth
- Take appropriate radiographs to confirm the position of any supernumerary, incisor crown, root anomalies, or any other abnormalities
- If there are positive finding at this stage, it is usually prudent to refer the patient for a specialist opinion. This may include:
  - removing any retained primary incisors or erupted supernumaries that may be impeding eruption of a permanent incisor – monitor closely and maintain space if the permanent incisor still fails to erupt soon thereafter

  or

  - referring the patient for surgical extraction of any supernumerary teeth, with or without exposure/removal of the unerupted incisor. In the meantime, maintain space using a simple sectional fixed appliance or removable space maintainer.

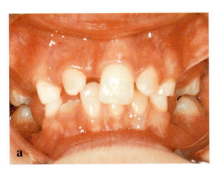
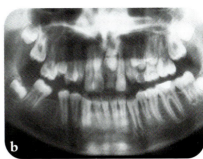
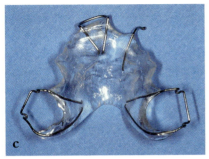
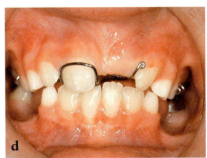
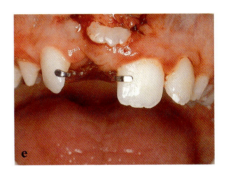

Fig 2-3 (a) Obvious asymmetry caused by an unerupted central incisor. (b) Radiograph of unerupted central incisor and retained primary incisor. (c) Design of a removable space maintainer to allow unimpeded eruption of an upper central incisor following removal of a supernumary. (d) Removable space maintainer in situ. (e) Surgical exposure of unerupted central incisor which failed to erupt even after removal of supernumary.

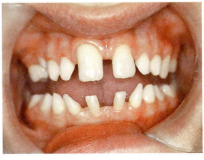

Fig 2-4 The typical appearance of hypodontia, with spacing and conical shaping of the anterior teeth that are present.

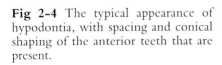

Congenitally missing teeth

Hypodontia – congenital absence of permanent teeth – is seen in between 4-6% of the population. The lower second premolars and the upper lateral incisors are the most commonly missing teeth, excluding third permanent molars. Management of hypodontia usually (Fig 2-4) warrants multidisciplinary specialist input. Therefore it is advisable to refer such patients for an early opinion regarding long-term treatment planning.

The following simple interventions can be considered:

• When second premolars are missing and the arch is either well-aligned or spaced, the second primary molar should be left *in situ* (assuming the tooth is of a reasonable prognosis). But where there is crowding, early removal of the second primary molar can be considered to relieve this crowding and thereby to facilitate space closure by mesial drift of the first permanent molar.

• When one, or both of the upper lateral incisors are missing in an uncrowded arch, the excess space is often distributed around the upper anterior segment. This space can be localised, to provide tooth-sized spaces for adhesive bridges, or closed completely and stabilised with a permanent retainer.

Ectopic teeth

The most common ectopic tooth is the maxillary canine, occurring in about 2% of the population. Of these, 85% are palatally placed and only 15% buccally placed relative to the line of the arch. The risk of impaction is higher where the lateral incisor is either peg-shaped or missing: the lateral incisor root is known to guide the canine into its appropriate place. One of the most important aspects of orthodontic screening is the locating of unerupted maxillary canines (Fig 2-5a, b). An impacted canine can resorb the adjacent lateral incisor root, and occasionally even the central incisor root. This can have a dramatic effect on the long-term prognosis of these teeth. It is imperative, therefore, to closely monitor for potential ectopic eruption of maxillary canines and to take appropriate action as suggested below:

• Palpate for the maxillary canines in the buccal sulcus from the age of nine years

• Check for mobility of the primary canines as an indication of the eruption of the permanent successor

• Where there is doubt as to the position of the canine, a radiographic assessment should be made. A periapical radiograph should reveal if the root of the primary canine is resorbing normally or if the canine follicle is enlarged. If the primary root is not resorbing, a further radiographic view is indicated to locate the permanent tooth (using the parallax technique)

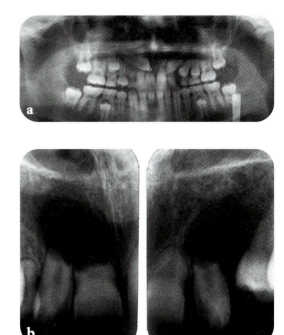

Fig 2-5 (a) Severe root resorption of the lateral and central incisors caused by the ectopic canines. (b) The radiographic appearance after the canines were inappropriately removed.

- If the permanent canine is found to be erupting in an ectopic path at an early stage (from about the age of 10), consider extracting the primary canine to encourage a more normal path of eruption. Extraction of the contralateral primary canine may also have to be undertaken to prevent centre-line shift
- There is a strong association between missing lateral incisors and palatally placed canines. Again, early extraction of primary canines may be advised, but in such cases an orthodontic opinion should be sought first.

O – Overjet

An increased overjet increases the likelihood of trauma to the upper permanent incisors. In fact, children with overjets of more than 10mm are more than twice as likely to traumatise their upper incisors than children with overjets of 5mm or less (Fig 2-6). The early reduction of a large overjet can reduce this risk of trauma, justifying early appliance therapy.

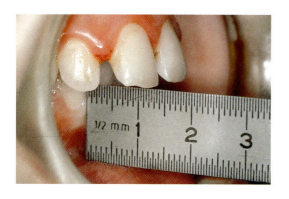

Fig 2-6 An overjet of this dimension more than doubles the risk of traumatic injury to the upper anterior teeth.

The reduction in overjet during the mixed dentition stage can often be accomplished using a functional appliance, although patient compliance with a functional appliance can be a problem. Functional appliances work by harnessing the forces generated by the masticatory and facial musculature to hold the mandible in a forward-postured position. The major limitations of these appliances are that they only work in growing children, and that they cannot treat irregularities of arch alignment, such as crowding. The goal of treatment is to reduce the overjet to normal within a six-month period, but prolonged night-time-only wear will be required. Treatment with a functional appliance may be a precursor to fixed appliances in the permanent dentition.

In other circumstances – for example, where an increased overjet is due simply to very proclined upper incisors – a simple removable appliance may be indicated for correction. Compliance with a removable appliance is generally better than with a functional appliance. Good patient selection is the key to success.

C – Crossbites

Anterior cross-bites
These can develop in the mixed dentition stage and can often be corrected with removable appliances in a relatively short time (10-12 weeks), with good compliance (Fig 2-7a, b). It is important to correct anterior crossbites for the following reasons:
- to avoid adjacent teeth also erupting into cross-bite
- to prevent trauma to the lower incisors
- to prevent the development of occlusal dysfunction
- to prevent the development of temporomandibular joint problems.

The occlusion is favourable for correction if:
- the affected tooth, or teeth are palatally inclined
- there is sufficient space to procline the teeth
- there is not an underlying severe Class III skeletal relationship
- there will be an adequate post-treatment overbite for the situation to be stable.

In terms of appliance design, an upper removable appliance is usually recommended. The appliance should incorporate:
- enough posterior capping to free the occlusion
- good retention using Adams clasps and a Southend clasp anteriorly (three-point fixation)
- Z-springs as the active component
- a mid-line screw for arch expansion if space is required to push the anterior tooth/teeth over the bite.

Posterior cross-bites
These may be either unilateral or bilateral, and with or without displacement on closure (Fig 2-8). They may also be seen in conjunction with a digit-sucking habit. Except in unusual circumstances, only unilateral cross-bites with displacement need active treatment, as these usually involve the displacement of a whole quadrant. The most common method of treatment is expansion of the upper arch to remove the initial cusp-to-cusp contact, using:
- an upper removable appliance with a mid-line screw that is turned regularly, or
- a quad-helix appliance fixed to bands on the upper first permanent molars.

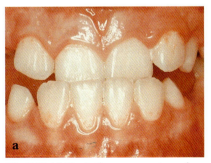
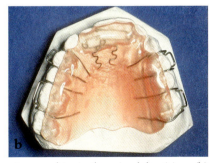

Fig 2-7 (a) Typical representation of an anterior crossbite in the mixed dentition. (b) Removable appliance design to correct an anterior crossbite. Note the retention and the posterior capping to 'free' the occlusion.

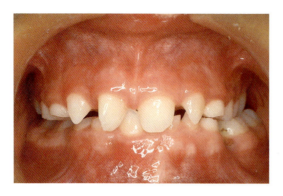

Fig 2-8 Posterior crossbite, in addition to spaced and rotated anterior teeth.

It is currently advised that there is little advantage to be gained in treating cross-bites in the primary dentition. Active treatment should usually be post-poned until the mixed dentition stage.

D – Displacement (of Contact Points)

Displacement of contact points most commonly results from crowding. This can present in the primary dentition, where its presence is a strong predic-tor of permanent dentition-crowding. When a child has crowding, the extraction of posterior primary teeth will, in general, tend to make this worse by allowing the mesial drifting of teeth distal to the extraction site (Fig 2-9). There tends to be little movement of primary anterior teeth after extraction unless the dentition was very crowded to start with. In general, decisions about extractions to relieve crowding in the permanent dentition should be left at least until the eruption of the permanent incisors is complete at around nine years of age.

The terms balancing and compensating extractions are widely used, but sometimes give rise to confusion. Balancing an extraction means remov-ing the contralateral tooth in the same arch, whereas compensating extrac-tions refers to the removal of the equivalent tooth in the opposing arch. As far as the primary dentition is concerned, there is rarely a need to com-pensate extractions. In addition, balancing extractions are indicated only for primary canines and first primary molars when the primary dentition is crowded. Such extractions may prevent a centre-line shift, which may create problems in the future and can be difficult to correct. Guidance on balancing and compensating first permanent molar extractions is given in Table 2-3.

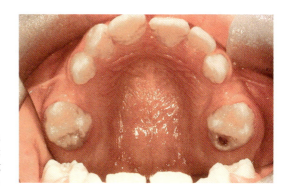

Fig 2-9 Marked space loss due to mesial drifting of first permanent molars following extraction of primary molars.

O – Overbite

An increased overbite in the primary dentition or when the permanent central incisors first erupt tends to improve spontaneously and is often of little consequence. An increased overbite in the permanent dentition may arise in a skeletal Class II malocclusion because of over-eruption of the incisors in the absence of incisal contact. In the mixed dentition phase such increased overbites are sometimes treated using a removable appliance with an anterior bite plane. The use of functional appliances has increased significantly in popularity over the past few years and may, in selected cases, be the preferred option. The indications for functional appliance therapy are as follows:
- mild crowding (1-4mm)
- growing patient
- Class II skeletal malocclusion, mostly due to mandibular retrognathism
- normal to low Frankfort Mandibular Plane Angle.

O – Others

Space maintenance
Remaining teeth will drift mesially into an extraction space, in particular in the upper arch, and where there is pre-existing crowding. It is particularly important that this space loss is prevented following the loss of a second primary molar or a permanent upper incisor; and where crowding is of such severity that extractions will produce only just enough space for arch alignment. Where any of these situations occur, the use of a space maintainer may be indicated (Figs 2-10 and 2-11). A simple acrylic appliance with Adams clasps and a suitably extended baseplate may be used. In the lower arch a lingual bar retained by bands on the first permanent molars

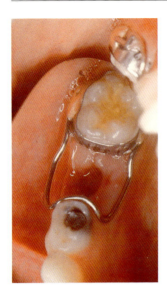

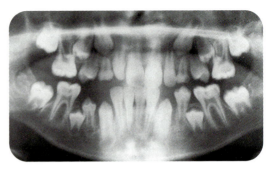

Fig 2-10 (left) An example of a fixed space maintainer, fitted after the extraction of a second primary molar to prevent mesial drifting of the first permanent molar.

Fig 2-11 (top) Almost complete space closure by the first permanent molars, with resulting impaction of the second premolars in all four quadrants.

is best tolerated. The long-term benefits of a space maintainer must be carefully weighed up against oral hygiene and increased caries risk for the patient. Furthermore, children who have required multiple extractions of primary molars may not be the most compliant patients for the provision of space maintainers.

Digit-sucking habits
Thumb- and finger-sucking habits persisting into the mixed dentition can cause an anterior open bite, an increased overjet or a unilateral posterior crossbite with mandibular displacement. Most children grow out of thumb-sucking by the age of 10, when an anterior open bite may resolve spontaneously. Occasionally, however, the tongue will have adapted to the open bite and contact the lower lip to make an anterior seal during swallowing. In such circumstances appliance therapy is usually required to correct the increased overjet or unilateral crossbite.

There are a number of different 'habit-breaking' appliances available, but their use is indicated only occasionally, as many children abandon the habit spontaneously and any occlusal discrepancies are usually relatively easy to correct.

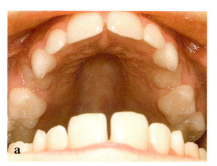 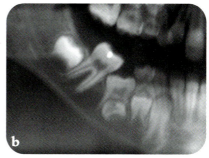

Fig 2-12 (a) Infraoccluded ('submerging') first primary molars. (b) Severe infraocclusion of second primary molar, even with developing second premolar present.

Infraocclusion

Previously described as submerged teeth, occasionally one, or more of the primary molars fail to maintain their appropriate position within the developing alveolus. It therefore appears to sink into the alveolar ridge and may eventually become buried. The condition is fairly common (affecting about 11% of primary molars) and most frequently involves lower first primary molars (Fig 2-12a, b). Approximately 99% of infraoccluded primary molars with a permanent successor exfoliate normally. Therefore no intervention is typically indicated, and the teeth can simply be kept under review. Where there is no successor and infraocclusion is severe, early extraction may be indicated before a surgical approach becomes necessary. In some cases, where space loss has occurred in the region of the infraoccluded tooth, it may be helpful to first recreate space orthodontically to facilitate tooth removal.

Midline diastema

Spacing and irregularity of the permanent incisors during the eruptive process is so common it should be regarded as normal, and parents should be reassured that much of the apparent malocclusion will correct spontaneously. Occasionally, however, an upper diastema may be related to the presence of a mid-line supernumerary tooth (a mesiodens), which should be identified radiographically and usually removed. The role of a thick labial frenum in producing a median diastema is less clear (Fig 2-13). It is generally recommended that the decision to undertake a fraenectomy is postponed until the active phase of orthodontic treatment.

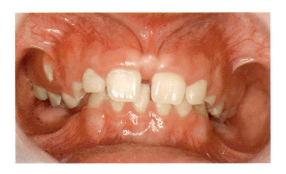

Fig 2-13 Midline diastema with large fleshy fraenal attachment.

The Dilemma of the First Permanent Molars

One of the most common interceptive decisions to be made in Paediatric Dentistry is whether or not to extract some, or all of the first permanent molars. While these teeth have been described as the 'cornerstone' of the occlusion, they are the permanent teeth most frequently affected by dental caries as a consequence of their prolonged exposure to the oral environment. In addition, they are affected by developmental defects more commonly than any other teeth, and the restoration of affected teeth is undoubtedly challenging, due in part to the difficulties of isolation, achieving anaesthesia, and of relatively poor patient compliance in the six- to seven-year-old age group. In cases where a first permanent molar is of extremely poor prognosis, the decision to extract may be a foregone conclusion. Decisions are not always so simple, however, and a number of factors have to be taken into account when assessing first permanent molars for extraction (Table 2-3).

The Occlusion
It is self-evident that extractions should be avoided if at all possible in a spaced dentition. The extraction of a first permanent molar creates a lot of space (approximately 10mm) in the posterior segment, and this is undesirable where there is already spacing in the dentition. Upper anterior crowding will not be relieved by the extraction of first permanent molars, although lower anterior crowding may improve marginally.

Where there has been early loss of the primary molars, in particular the second primary molar, there is often mesial drifting of the first permanent molar. This results in a shortage of space for the erupting premolars, and the extraction of one or two first permanent molars may be indicated to relieve this in the medium term. In some circumstances, premolar extractions are also required at a later stage.

38

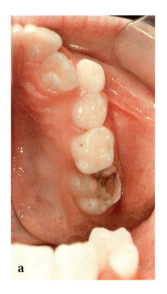

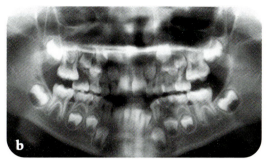

Fig 2-14 (a) Hypoplastic upper first permanent molar of poor long-term prognosis. (b) The radiographic appearance of the same molar: note the resorption of the upper second primary molars by the upper first permanent molars.

The Prognosis of the Teeth

Although dental caries rates have fallen in some countries, many children still have first permanent molars of doubtful prognosis by the age of eight or nine years. Where caries is extensive - that is, extending more than two-thirds of the way through dentine - the successful long-term restoration of the tooth is questionable. Cervical caries on the lingual surface of the lower first permanent molar or the buccal surface of the upper molar are also indicative of a poor prognosis. In addition, where caries has extended subgingivally in a young patient the tooth may be extremely difficult to restore. Pinned restorations are largely outdated and, in any case, contraindicated in young patients, given the relatively large size of the pulp. Bonded amalgams or preformed metal crowns are an alternative.

Over the past five to 10 years there has been a significant increase in the number of patients being identified with enamel defects, including hypoplasia and hypomineralisation (Fig 2-14a, b). Where one or more of the first permanent molars is affected by enamel defects, the outlook for all four teeth should be considered, and any extractions should be performed at the appropriate developmental stage.

'Balancing' and 'compensating' extractions need to be considered when contemplating the removal of first permanent molars. For guidelines on when

Table 2-3 **Guidelines on when to balance and when to compensate first permanent molar extractions in the mixed dentition**

Tooth/ Teeth Requiring Extraction (ISO no)	Clinical Situation 1	Clinical Situation 2	Clinical Situation 3	Clinical Situation 4
	Class I, no crowding/ mild crowding, OJ< 3mm, no reduction required, inadequate space for canines and premolars	*Class I, no crowding/ mild spacing; OJ<3mm no reduction re-quired, no incisor crowding, excess space*	*Class II, OJ>3mm, maxillary incisor crowding; inadequate space for premolars*	*Class III, reverse overjet*
36 or 46	Extract opposing maxillary FPM, usually also extract FPMs on other side, unless removal of a premolar would achieve a better result	Extract opposing maxillary FPM, do not extract FPMs on other side unless prognosis is poor	Either extract opposing FPM, or postpone until maxillary SPM erupts. Usually also extract FPM on the other side, unless removal of premolar would give better result	Restore opposing FPM if possible. Do not extract mandibular FPM on other side unless prognosis is poor and canines/ premolars are crowded

Tooth/ Teeth Requiring Extraction (ISO no)	Clinical Situation 1	Clinical Situation 2	Clinical Situation 3	Clinical Situation 4
36 or 46	Extract both opposing FPMs	*As for clinical situation 1*	*As above*	*As above*
16 or 26	Do not extract opposing mandibular FPM, unless its prognosis is poor	*As for clinical situation 1*	*As for clinical situation 1*	Do not extract maxillary FPM on other side unless its prognosis is poor
16 *and* 26	Do not extract opposing mandibular FPM, unless its prognosis is poor	*As for clinical situation 1*	*As for clinical situation 1*	Do not extract maxillary FPM unless its prognosis is poor

★ FPM = first permanent molar SPM = second permanent molar OJ = overjet

to balance and when to compensate, see Table 2-3. In general, balancing is not indicated for first permanent molars if the contralateral tooth is of good prognosis, as a centre-line shift is unlikely to develop. Compensation (ie, the extraction of the opposing tooth) is, however, often indicated to prevent over-eruption and possible impediment of desired mesial movement of the erupting second permanent molar.

The Patient's Compliance with Treatment

The ability of a young patient to accept dental treatment is a key consideration when treatment planning. If the patient is unable to cope with block anaesthesia, rubber dam, high-volume suction, matrix band placement - to give just some examples - then the options for treatment planning are reduced. There may be time available to undertake a programme of acclimatisation and desensitisation, and there may be sedation facilities close to hand. Equally, however, there may be no realistic alternative to arranging a general anaesthetic for first permanent molar extractions in, for example, a nervous eight-year-old.

The Wishes of the Parent and Patient

The principle of consent to treatment is well established, but it can be complicated when the wishes of a child patient are in conflict with those of the parent. Clearly it is helpful if any divergent opinions can be 'harmonised' by education and explanation of options and consequences, but occasionally this is not possible. There are some regional differences in legislation relating to child consent for medical and dental treatment. Where there are conflicts, it is important to understand the local procedures. A detailed discussion of consent is beyond the scope of this text, but an appropriate reference is given at the end of this chapter.

Timing of Extractions

It is well documented that the ideal time to extract first permanent molars is when the inter-radicular crescent of the root appears radiographically on the lower second permanent molar, corresponding to a 'dental age' of around nine years four months. Timing of extractions in the lower arch is more critical than for the upper arch. If the first permanent molar is extracted too early, the second premolar may have a tendency to migrate distally and erupt, leaving a space between the premolars. If the first permanent molar is extracted too late, the second permanent molar may not move sufficiently to close the space or may tip rather than undergo any bodily movement at all (Figs 2-15a, b and 2-16a, b). The major consideration in the upper arch is the rapidity with which space closure will occur

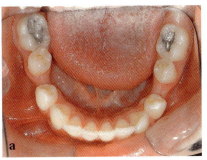
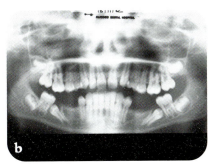

Fig 2-15 (a) First permanent molars were extracted too early, and the second premolars have drifted distally until contacting the second permanent molars. (b) Lower first molars extracted very early, upper first permanent molars still in situ. Impaction of the unerupted lower second premolars.

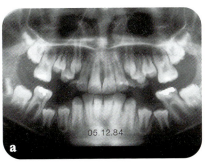
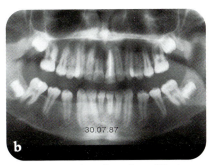

Fig 2-16 (a) Ideal timing of extraction of first permanent molars: furcation of the lower second permanent molar developing. (b) Spontaneous alignment of the teeth three years later.

following extractions. Where retention of space is critical, it is advisable to fit a space maintainer before carrying out extractions.

It may be considered, after reading this section, that extraction of first permanent molars is an excellent treatment option. It should be realised, however, that the removal of these key teeth from the dental arches is almost always a compromise that usually prolongs or otherwise complicates orthodontic treatment. Furthermore, loss of first permanent molars may result in poor contact areas between second premolars and second permanent molars and may delay interceptive orthodontic treatment, given the absence of suitable teeth for retention of a removable appliance.

Recommended Reading

Davies SJ, Gray RJ, Mackie IC. Good occlusal practice in children's dentistry. British Dental Journal 2001;191:655-659.

Gill DS, Lee RT, Tredwin CJ. Treatment planning for the loss of first permanent molars. Dental Update 2001;28:304-308.

Kirschen R. Orthodontic clinical screening in less than one minute. British Dental Journal 1998;185:224-226.

Leighton BC. The value of prophesy in orthodontics. Dental Practice 1971;21:359-372.

Richardson A. Interceptive Orthodontics. London: BDA Publications, 1999.

Sandler PJ, Atkinson R, Murray AM. For four sixes. American Journal of Dentofacial Orthopaedics 2000;117:418-34.

Chapter 3
Planning for Prevention

Aim

This chapter aims to review a range of preventive therapies that may be considered for the young patient. We hope to illustrate how every child should have a personalised preventive programme that reflects their individual social, medical and dental needs.

Outcomes

On reading this chapter, the practitioner will have gained a comprehensive understanding of the following preventive regimens:
- dietary advice
- antimicrobial therapy
- oral hygiene instruction
- prescribing fluoride
- fissure sealing
- provision of mouthguards.

Introduction

Why Prevention?
- Prevention of disease initiation or progression is fundamental to any community-based or personalised health programme.
- A preventive approach will contribute to overall health gain as well as having psychological and economical advantages.
- Systematic reviews have confirmed the effectiveness of various preventive dental interventions (see http://www.cochrane-oral.man.ac.uk).

The Problems with Prevention
Many dental problems are preventable, yet they continue to comprise most of everyday practice. Somewhere along the line, the preventive 'message' is failing, possibly because:
- Some preventive strategies demand patient or parent compliance; although advice is given, there is no guarantee that the patient/parent will act on it.

- Imparting knowledge may result in a change in attitude, but ultimately a change in behaviour may be outside the patient's control, given the complex interaction of relevant social and environmental factors.

Nonetheless, we are ethically obliged to provide realistic preventive advice, albeit that we sometimes feel we are banging our head against the surgery wall.

Whose Responsibility is it?

Recent years have seen radical changes in the delivery of dental care and the way in which dental services are funded. We now work as part of a dental team, comprising dentists, dental health educators, hygienists and therapists, dental nurses and dental technicians. Prevention may be seen increasingly as something prescribed by the dentist, but implemented by another member of the dental team (Fig 3-1).

What are we Trying to Prevent?

It is worth clarifying what conditions we are trying to prevent in young patients. These conditions include:
- dental caries (not just the initiation of a lesion but its progression)
- dental erosion
- gingival and periodontal disease
- dental trauma

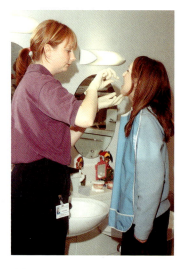

Fig 3-1 Dental nurse giving oral hygiene instruction.

Where does Prevention come in a Treatment Plan?

Prevention cannot be started soon enough. Ideally, parents should be encouraged to bring their children to the surgery from the age of around six months. This will ensure that appropriate oral hygiene and dietary advice are given before problems arise.

Prevention must be at the heart of any treatment plan. It usually forms the first phase of treatment for the following reasons:

- It frequently ties in with a behaviour-management strategy. Oral hygiene instruction, topical fluoride application and fissure-sealant placement are confidence- and trust-building steps. These steps lead to a more cooperative and happy patient during the latter, and more demanding, stages of a treatment plan.
- If the cause of an existing or potential dental problem is not identified and addressed, operator and patient time will be wasted. Caries is the obvious example: if the diet is not controlled and fluoride and fissure sealants applied, new cavities will continue to appear at each visit.

Prevention should not, however, be restricted to the first visit. It should continue throughout the child's course of treatment with regular reinforcement and re-assessment of need.

'Tailor-Made' Prevention

Preventive strategies should be individualised, based on an assessment of each child's risk of caries, erosion, gingival and periodontal disease and trauma. Some of the social, medical and dental considerations that might influence a preventive treatment plan are highlighted in Table 3-1.

Dietary Advice

Diet analysis and advice are pivotal in the prevention of caries and tooth erosion in young patients. Dietary education probably represents the most challenging part of the preventive repertoire. Although we may give helpful advice, we cannot be sure that patients will act on it. Despite the recognised limitations of diet histories, it is still helpful to ask selected children and their parents to produce a three-day (including one weekend day) written record of their entire food and drink consumption. It is then possible to:

- highlight the cariogenic or erosive items
- provide simple and positive suggestions for reducing their frequency of intake.

Table 3-1 **Patient variables that may influence a preventive strategy**

Patient Variable	Considerations for Prevention
Social factors	
Irregular attender	• likely to have poor compliance with preventive advice – best not to send off with a bottle of fluoride tablets
Low socio-economic group	• likely to have high caries rates • recommend high fluoride-containing toothpaste • consider fissure sealants • may be unable to afford recommended oral hygiene aids
Minority ethnic groups	• high primary dentition caries rates in many groups • dietary advice may be complicated owing to language difficulties or uncertainty about the cariogenic potential of certain food and drink
Medical factors	
Congenital heart defects	• children at risk of infective endocarditis should receive intense preventive care
Oncology patients	• patients may become immunocompromised during chemotherapy – it is essential to maintain oral health and to instigate a rigorous preventive programme to reduce the risk of a mid-treatment dental crisis
Haematological disorders	• early prevention should ensure that extractions due to caries are avoided

Special needs/learning disability	• prevention must take priority, especially as this may be the only form of treatment the patient will tolerate • advice may have to be given to carers if the child is not in the home environment
On long term medication	• try to ensure that medications are sugar-free

Dental factors

Rampant caries	• this may be 'bottle caries' in the younger patient or rapidly progressive lesions in a teenager. Either way, before any invasive treatment is instigated (unless for pain relief) invest some time in formulating a sound preventive programme
Erosion	• diagnose early and give appropriate advice – be alert to a possible underlying eating disorder in teenagers, in particular girls • consider fissure-sealing exposed dentine • prescribe professional or patient-applied topical fluoride
Low salivary flow	• in cases of rampant caries consider whether an abnormally low salivary flow may be an exacerbating factor; if so, consider referral, saliva substitutes, fluoride rinses and sugar-free chewing gum
Orthodontic patients	• oral hygiene and dietary practices must be optimal before, and during orthodontic treatment • recommend 0.05% fluoride rinses throughout treatment • identify children with an increased overjet, as they are more prone to trauma, and consider mouthguards for sports or early interceptive treatment to reduce the over-jet

Dental anomalies	• Amelogenesis imperfecta patients may need extra help with oral hygiene given dental sensitivity and plaque accumulation on pitted/grooved enamel • fissure-seal deep cingulum pits or dens-in-dente type teeth on eruption to prevent possible pulpal contamination • instigate a rigorous preventive programme for hypodontia patients
Periodontal disease	• the initiation of aggressive periodontal disease in children may not be preventable, but its progression can be limited by early diagnosis and appropriate referral

The Dos and Don'ts of Dietary Advice

3 **Do**	5 **Don't**
3 Keep it simple (no more than three points) and write advice down for the patient 3 Suggest alternatives 3 Repeat dietary records to check for improvements 3 Make patients aware of 'toothfriendly' sugar-free products (bearing in mind they are not recommended for the very young, given their possible gastrointestinal side-effects)	5 Do not be judgemental 5 Do not be too negative: try to find at least one good point to comment on 5 Don't be unrealistic – we all eat sweets on occasions

Although specific dietary recommendations to prevent caries and erosion prevention are considered separately in the sections below, it is not uncommon for patients to demonstrate the tell-tale signs of a diet that is both cariogenic and acidogenic (Fig 3-2). As a consequence, dietary advice may need to address various aspects of prevention.

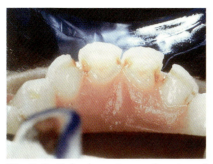

Fig 3-2 Palatal erosion and caries of upper primary incisors.

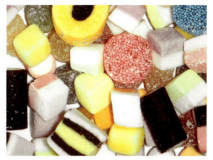

Fig 3-3 Chocolate would be preferable to chewy sweets.

Dietary Advice for Dental Caries

The aetiology of dental caries is multifactorial, but the major culprits are non-milk extrinsic ('free') sugars (Table 3-2). It is essential to reduce both the overall amount and frequency of intake of these sugars, both for dental health and overall health. Milk sugars (lactose) and intrinsic sugars (found in fruit and vegetables) have not been implicated in dental caries. Caries may, however, result from prolonged, on-demand breast-feeding or bottle-feeding at night.

Dietary Advice for Erosion

Tooth tissue loss, as a consequence of erosion, has become a common finding in young patients (Fig 3-4).

Following a diagnosis of erosion, the first priority is to identify and eliminate the cause to limit further tissue loss (Table 3-3).

Erosion is caused by acids from an intrinsic or extrinsic source. Intrinsic acids, from the stomach, may enter the mouth as a result of gastro-oesophageal reflux (common in children with neuromuscular problems, such as cerebral palsy), vomiting, or rumination. If any of these problems are suspected, a medical referral may be necessary. The most common source of extrinsic acids comes from drinks, including:
- fresh fruit juices
- fruit-flavoured drinks
- carbonated drinks.

Table 3-2 **Dietary advice for the prevention of dental caries**

Key Points	Other Comments
• Recommend safe snacks	fruit, bread, meat, cheese, plain crisps, nuts (older children only), sugar-free chewing gum
• Recommend safe drinks	water, plain milk, sugarless tea
• Avoid use of sweetened drinks in bottle or feeder cup	if a habit is already established try to progressively dilute soft drink with water until the child is practically drinking water only
• Discourage prolonged 'on-demand' breast-feeding	a controversial area, but breast milk has a higher lactose content than cow's milk and may be implicated in caries
• Try to limit confectionary to mealtimes or one day a week	and brush teeth afterwards
• Ban chewy or boiled sweets	chocolate is preferred to packets of hard or chewy sweets, which are usually eaten over a longer period of time
• Watch out for those 'hidden' sugars	sugars are present in flavoured crisps, fruit yoghurts and dried fruits, which may be perceived as healthy snacks

Other dietary sources of acids include:
- citrus fruits
- yoghurts
- pickled/vinegary foods
- chewable vitamin C tablets.

Table 3-3 **Dietary advice for the prevention of dental erosion**

- Limit erosive drinks to no more than once a day, ideally with a meal

- Follow an erosive attack with a drink of water or alkaline food, such as cheese

- Don't keep drinks in mouth for a prolonged period and try to drink quickly, possibly using a straw

- Refrain from brushing teeth for one hour after an erosive attack

- Advocate sugar-free chewing gum to stimulate salivary flow

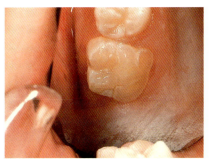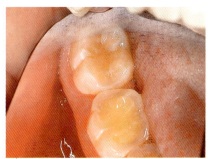

Fig 3-4 Severe erosion of first permanent molars in a 12-year-old boy.

Tip: In cases where drinks are implicated it is worth checking whether the child practises an abnormal drinking habit, such as swishing or frothing their drink before swallowing, as this can compound the erosive effect.

A useful educational aid is a supply of litmus strips (Fig 3-5). Patients are asked to bring along their favourite beverage and watch the colour of the strip change according to the acidity of the drink. Although the titratable acidity (amount of sodium hydroxide required to neutralise a solution) is a more accurate determinant of erosive potential than pH *per se*, the chemistry may be beyond the understanding of most patients, and a simpler message will suffice.

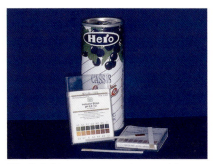

Fig 3-5 Litmus paper strips provide useful educational aids to demonstrate the erosive potential of drinks.

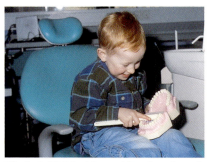

Fig 3-6 Child with toothbrush and tooth models.

Antimicrobial Therapy

In recent years more attention has been paid to the treatment of caries as an 'infectious disease'. There is now growing evidence to support the use of antimicrobial agents in caries prophylaxis. Chlorhexidine is the most studied and potent chemoprophylactic agent, exerting both a bacteriocidal and bacteriostatic effect. It can be used as a mouthwash, gel or varnish to reduce numbers of *Staphylococcus mutans* in plaque and saliva. It may be employed on a long-term basis, in conjunction with other preventive measures and in individuals with a high caries risk, although definitive clinical evidence for the effectiveness of this approach is still lacking.

Oral Hygiene Matters

The Scale of the Problem

- Plaque-induced gingivitis is common in children. Chronic marginal gingivitis is seen in about 25% of five-year-olds, 60% of nine-year-olds, and shows a peak incidence around the time of puberty (attributed to changing circulatory hormonal levels).
- Periodontal disease is relatively rare in young patients. However, chronic adult periodontal disease starts during early teenage years, with about 10% of British 15-year-olds showing 1-2mm of attachment loss.

A loss of periodontal attachment before the age of nine years is very unusual, and any rapidly progressive attachment loss warrants careful investigation.

Why Should Children Brush their Teeth?
- To develop good habits for the future (Fig 3-6).
- To prevent the development of plaque-induced gingival inflammation and other progressive gingival or periodontal diseases.
- To reduce caries initiation or progression by the application of a fluoridated toothpaste (via a toothbrush).
- To facilitate any restorative treatment, which is considerably more successful in the absence of inflamed and bleeding gums.
- To reduce the incidence of unsightly demineralised lesions during any orthodontic treatment.

Practical Instruction
Achieving optimal oral cleanliness should be a priority in any treatment plan. Indeed, treatments such as orthodontics and the provision of a laboratory-made prosthesis should be postponed until oral hygiene standards are acceptable.
- Oral hygiene instruction needs to be individualised according to specific patient factors, including age, manual dexterity, medical status, learning ability and the presence of any specific gingival or periodontal problems.
- Parents should instigate oral hygiene measures as soon as the child's primary incisors erupt.
- It is generally recommended that parents continue to brush their child's teeth until the age of at least six years (or long-term for children with special needs).
- Parents should be advised to use a small soft toothbrush and a smear of children's toothpaste.
- The dentist should demonstrate that the best access for toothbrushing is achieved by standing/sitting behind the child rather than approaching them from the front.
- The brushing technique adopted is not critical, as long as all the plaque is removed.
- In patients with high disease levels mechanical cleaning alone may not be sufficient to remove bacterial infection and should be supported by an antibacterial regime, such as a mouthwash.

Which Toothbrush?
No single toothbrush design has been shown to be more effective than any other, although it is important to ensure that the size is appropriate for the child's mouth (Fig 3-7). Specially designed toothbrushes, such as bottle brushes and single-tufted brushes are usually necessary for optimum plaque

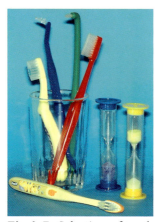

Fig 3-7 Selection of tooth brushes for the young patient.

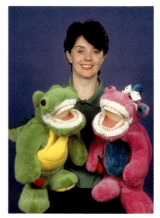

Fig 3-8 Hand puppets may help give oral hygiene instruction to young children.

control in patients wearing fixed orthodontic appliances. Specific instruction should be given to these patients.

Parents frequently ask whether an electric toothbrush offers any advantage to a manual toothbrush. Studies have suggested that powered toothbrushes with a rotation oscillation action may achieve slightly better plaque removal than manual brushes. In addition, children tend to like them, parents find them easier to use and in nervous children they may be a useful precursor to the introduction of the slow handpiece.

Oral Hygiene Aids
A number of aids can enhance oral hygiene instruction (Fig 3-8):
- Study models and spare toothbrushes are useful for demonstrating tooth-brushing techniques.
- Disclosing solutions and tablets (containing erythrocyin dyes) are also good for checking tooth-brushing efficacy at home and in the surgery, and their use is generally viewed as a fun activity (Fig 3-9).
- Motivated (or desperate) parents may consider placing a timer in the bathroom to ensure that children spend longer than 10 seconds brushing their teeth.
- Flossing demands a high level of manual dexterity and motivation and is not usually advised for young children. It may, however, be recommended for teenagers with early interstitial lesions or who have an adhesive bridge.

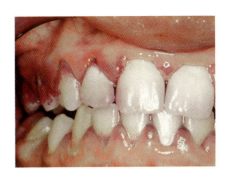

Fig 3-9 Disclosed teeth in a 12-year-old boy showing plaque accumulation on upper right premolars.

Monitoring Oral Hygiene

Plaque indices may be employed to provide a more objective assessment of oral cleanliness over consecutive visits. A very simple index is shown in Fig 3-10. This index involves an estimation of the amount of disclosed plaque on six key teeth.

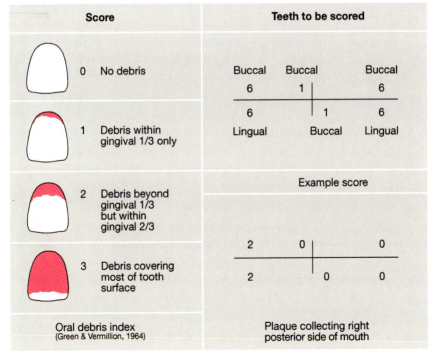

Fig 3-10 Objective approach for evaluation of oral cleanliness.

Specific Gingival and Periodontal Problems

Consideration of the spectrum of gingival and periodontal problems seen in children is beyond the scope of this book (Fig 3-11). Suggestions for further reading are given at the end of the chapter. The main point to stress is that early onset and aggressive loss of periodontal attachment warrants specialist referral, in particular as it may be an indicator of a serious underlying disease. The types of gingival and periodontal conditions seen in children and suggested courses of action are summarised in Table 3-4.

Table 3-4 **Management of gingival and periodontal conditions in children**

Diagnosis	Presentation	Suggested Action
Plaque-induced chronic marginal gingivitis	• painless, red, swollen, bleeding gums	• prophylaxis and OHI
Gingival hyperplasia (drug-induced)	• painless pink fibrous enlarged gingivae • interdental papillae may appear nodular • may have superimposed plaque-induced marginal gingivitis	• meticulous oral hygiene needed • use of single-tufted toothbrushes • chlorhexidine solution can be applied to deep pockets via a blunt needle and syringe • discuss possibility of changing medication with patient's paediatrician
Acute herpetic gingivostomatitis	• usually affects younger children (two to five years of age) • malaise • pyrexia • drooling • loss of appetite • cervical lymphadenopathy • initially multiple	• supportive advice, fluids, bland diet, paracetamol, bed rest • soft toothbrush/sponges soaked in chlorhexidine • review (condition is self-limiting after 10–14 days) • systemic antivirals (acyclovir) are indicated

Diagnosis	Presentation	Suggested Action
	vesicles along the buccal gingivae, tongue, palate or lips that rapidly rupture, leaving small ulcers • spontaneous oral bleeding may occur	in immunosupressed patients only on discussion with their paediatrician
Self-induced gingival injury (gingivitis artefacta)	• uncommon • may present with localised severe loss of supporting tissues and exposed roots • may be due to pre-existing source of irritation, habit, or underlying psychological problem	• if caused by known habit (for instance, pencil-chewing) advise and monitor • if self-harm persists with denial of injury, a psychiatric referral may be indicated
Localised gingival and periodontal recession (Stillman's cleft)	• usually gingival recession is limited to labial surface of a lower incisor and may be associated with occlusal trauma, crowding, poor oral hygiene or a high fraenal attachment	• OHI and professional scaling • chlorhexidine application • eliminate occlusal trauma • may require orthodontic treatment
Prepubertal periodontitis	• may be localised or generalised severe loss of supporting tissues, with premature exfoliation of primary teeth • generalised type presents	• supportive OH measures • antibiotics • referral to specialist for investigation of possible underlying immunological problem

Diagnosis	Presentation	Suggested Action
	with fiery red gingivae that may bleed spontaneously	• in generalised cases full dental clearances under antibiotic cover may be necessary
Juvenile periodontitis	• may be localised or generalised • rapid loss of supporting tissues initially affects permanent incisors and first permanent molars; may present with drifting or mobile teeth • gingivae not usually inflamed • more common in Black African or Asian teenage girls	• regular scaling, root planing, OHI • antibiotics • antiplaque agents • consider referral for specialist treatment

★ OH = oral hygiene
  OHI = oral hygiene instruction

Fluoride: Friend or Foe?

Despite a wealth of evidence to support the anticaries effects of fluoride, considerable opposition still remains to its therapeutic use - in particular, in public water supplies. Excessive fluoride intake at a young age can lead to the development of fluoride-induced enamel defects. There is therefore an onus on the dental profession to prescribe fluoride judiciously, carefully weighing up the risk of dental fluorosis against caries-prevention benefits.

Fluoride Dietary Supplements

If taken at an appropriate stage of dental development, systemic fluoride effects a change in enamel structure, increasing its resistance to acid demineralisation. In the UK, fluoride supplements (sodium fluoride) are available as drops and tablets, available on prescription only. These supplements are recommended only for children with a high caries risk and where compliance is assured. There is considerable worldwide variation in both the dose

Table 3-5 **Recommended fluoride supplement dosages**

Age	Dose per Day	Comment
Six months to three years	0.25mg fluoride	• Before the age of six months, kidney function is not mature enough to cope with fluoride excretion • Some would delay fluoride supplements until the child is three years old, as permanent incisors have completed the 'critical' phase of enamel development by this time and cannot therefore develop any fluoride–induced opacities
Three to six years	0.5mg fluoride	• Tablets should be chewed to gain a topical as well as systemic effect
Over six years	1.0mg fluoride	• After the age of six years, systemic fluoride cannot affect developing enamel since, with exception of third permanent molars, it has already formed. However, tablets may still be indicated for their topical effect in those patients unable to use other topical fluoride preparations

and recommended age for fluoride supplementation for children. Recommendations issued by the British Society of Paediatric Dentistry (1996) are set out in Table 3-5.

Reported reductions in caries experience from dietary fluoride supplements vary widely, with most studies having been carried out several decades ago. Overall, a 40-80% reduction in caries may be expected in both dentitions when supplements are started by the age of two years.

The Dos and Don'ts of Fluoride Supplement Prescription

Do	Don't
Prescribe fluoride supplements only for children with a high caries experience in the early primary dentition (or where there is a known family history of caries) and for medically compromised children who are most at risk from the sequelae of dental caries	Do not prescribe fluoride supplements for children who are receiving fluoridated water supplies or fluoridated milk
Do tell parents to cease fluoride supplements temporarily when travelling to areas of unknown water fluoridation levels (it may take only one acute increase in plasma fluoride concentration to cause fluoride-induced opacities)	Do not prescribe supplements if there is a history of toothpaste-eating habits or if parental compliance is suspect
Do tell parents to give fluoride supplements at a different time to normal tooth-brushing to avoid a large surge in fluoride plasma concentration and to maximise the number of topical fluoride exposures	

Fluoridated Milk

Dentists should be proactive in encouraging their patients to accept fluoridated milk if such a scheme is available in their area (Fig 3-12). A number of regions have now implemented school fluoridated milk schemes. By 2004, about 16,000 primary school children were receiving fluoridated milk. Fol-

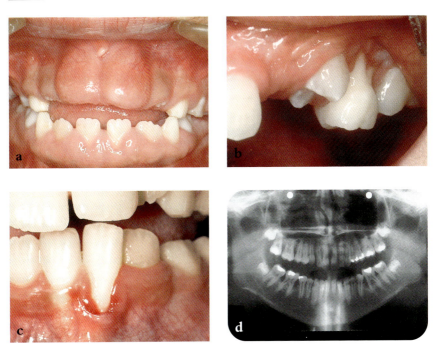

Fig 3-11 Some gingival and periodontal conditions seen in young patients. (a) Drug-induced gingival hyperplasia in a kidney transplant patient. (b) Self-inflicted gingival trauma with a lead pencil. (c) Localised gingival recession. (d) Marked bone loss around first permanent molars in a teenage girl with juvenile periodontitis.

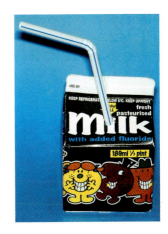

Fig 3-12 Fluoridated school milk.

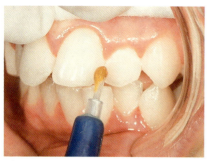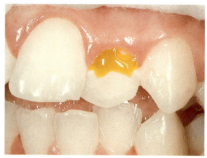

Fig 3-13 Fluoridated varnish application to an early carious 'white spot' lesion.

lowing written parental consent, 189ml cartons of milk containing 2.65ppm of sodium fluoride are provided in schools on a daily basis.

Worldwide studies have reported a 0-83% reduction in caries experience in the permanent dentition with fluoridated milk consumption.

Fluoridated Water

Implementation of new public water fluoridation schemes has made little progress in the UK over the past 30-40 years. Only 10% of the population currently receive a fluoridated water supply.

The York report, published in 2000, reviewed the world literature on the safety and efficacy of fluoridated water and reported a decrease of 2.2 in the mean number of decayed, missing or filled teeth.

Fluoridated Varnishes

Fluoridated varnishes are for topical application by dental professionals only (Fig 3-13). The extremely high fluoride concentration (Duraphat contains 22,600ppm) means that sparing application is recommended to avoid unpleasant gastrointestinal side- effects. Regular (three-monthly) applications of fluoride varnish may be effective in arresting early 'white spot' lesions. It may also be helpful in reversing the caries process in some cavitated lesions.

A recent Cochrane review concluded that regular fluoride varnish applications could reduce caries in the primary dentition by 33% and by 46% in the permanent dentition.

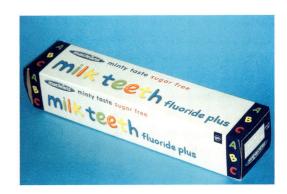

Fig 3-14 1,000ppm fluoridated toothpaste is recommended for young children with high caries risk.

Fluoride applications can be used as part of a behaviour management strategy as well as a preventive one: most small children (and nervous adolescents) will accept 'banana paint' on their teeth. The patient should be asked not to eat or drink for 30 minutes after the application. This maximises the uptake of fluoride ions into the tooth surface.

Fluoride Gels
Gels containing high levels of fluoride (12,300ppm) can be applied to teeth professionally by means of upper and lower trays. Care should be taken to avoid excessive fluoride ingestion, as this may result in gastrointestinal upset. This regimen has been shown to reduce caries incidence by about 20%.

Some fluoridated gels are also available for home use (Gel-Kam) and may be indicated for selected patients, including:
- those wearing overdentures or removable orthodontic appliances (the gel can be placed on the fitting surface of the appliance before insertion)
- children with severe erosion from an intrinsic acid source (the gel can be placed under protective mouthguards).

Fluoridated Toothpastes
The market for children's toothpastes has seen enormous growth over recent years. These products are essential for caries prevention (Fig 3-14).

Use of fluoridated toothpastes can effect a 24% reduction in caries in children's permanent teeth and a 37% reduction in primary dentition caries. The effectiveness is directly related to fluoride concentration, with an estimated 6% reduction in caries for every 500ppm increase in fluoride.

The Dos and Don'ts of Fluoride Toothpaste Usage for Children

3 Do	5 Don't
3 Use only a smear of toothpaste for young children (the under-twos reportedly ingest about 50% of the toothpaste they are given) 3 Brush twice daily 3 Brush last thing at night	5 Do not recommend a toothpaste containing more than 600ppm fluoride for children under six years unless assessed as high caries risk 5 Do not rinse after brushing (just spit)

It is important to consider caries risk when recommending the most appropriate toothpaste. For young patients determined as 'high risk', even the under-sixes should use a toothpaste containing higher fluoride levels (up to 1,000 ppm).

The Dos and Don'ts of Fluoride Rinses

3 Do	5 Don't
3 Recommend for patients wearing orthodontic appliances 3 Recommend for patients with multiple early lesions of caries after rinsing 3 Recommend for patients with a high previous caries experience 3 Recommend for patients with erosion 3 Recommend for medically compromised patients 3 Recommend rinsing at a different time to tooth-brushing in order to maintain high fluoride concentrations for a longer period of time 3 Recommend an alcohol-free fluoride rinse for children	5 Do not prescribe for the under-sixes, or anyone else who is unable to rinse and spit reliably 5 Do not eat or drink for 30 minutes after rising 5 Do not rinse with water after using the mouthwash

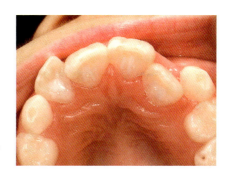

Fig 3-15 Opaque fissure sealant occluding deep palatal pits on upper incisors.

Fluoride Rinses

The daily use of a 0.05% sodium fluoride rinse (230ppm fluoride) can effect a 30% reduction in caries incidence.

Fissure Sealants

Fissure sealants have been around for about 50 years and form a valuable component of our preventive armamentarium (Fig 3-15). Fissure sealants reduce pit and fissure caries in permanent molars by between 46-71% in children at high risk of caries.

Sealants are easy to apply, yet just as easy to do badly. Sealants may, however, be expected to last three years in approximately 50% of cases. After placement of a sealant it is critical to review and maintain it at regular intervals. Early detection of stain penetration beneath a sealant indicates marginal failure and the need for replacement.

Who Should Have Sealants?

The following priority patient groups should be considered for fissure sealants:
- children with a history of caries in the primary dentition
- medically compromised children
- children with special needs, in particular those with a learning disability
- children with early occlusal caries in one or more first permanent molars
- erosion cases
- children with mildly hypoplastic molars
- children with teeth with particularly deep pits and fissures
- children who cannot maintain good levels of oral cleanliness.

When and What to Seal

In cases of high caries risk, permanent teeth should be sealed soon after eruption, providing that adequate isolation and moisture control can be achieved. Fissure sealants may, however, be considered at any time. For instance, they may be indicated in a teenager who has started to show early signs of caries since becoming acquainted with the vending machine at secondary school.

Although the occlusal surface of the permanent molar is a priority site for the application of a fissure sealant, there are other caries-prone sites that may also benefit from the protection of fissure sealants. These include:
- primary molars (sealants may be indicated to prevent the progression of very early occlusal lesions in young patients, although there is currently no data to support their effectiveness in the primary dentition)
- deep grooves present on the buccal surfaces of some molars
- deep cingulum pits present on the palatal aspect of upper anterior teeth
- exposed dentine with an underlying erosive aetiology
- exposed dentine in recently traumatised teeth (calcium hydroxide covered by a fissure sealant can provide a quick 'emergency' stopguard)
- sites of 'abnormal' tooth morphology, such as the deep fissures surrounding a talon cusp or over the communication to a suspected dens-in-dente.

Which Type of Sealant?

- Unfilled sealants tend to have better flow characteristics and are preferable on stained fissures to facilitate monitoring of any caries progression.
- Opaque or tinted sealants are easier to see, aiding initial placement and review.
- Fluoride-containing sealants have not been found to be of any therapeutic advantage and have been found to have poorer retention rates than conventional sealants.
- Fissure obliteration can also be achieved with glass-ionomer cements. Appropriate materials can be run into fissures as soon as the tooth erupts without the need for etching. Although retention rates are poor, they do provide an interim sealant until the tooth has fully erupted or patient compliance allows placement of a 'conventional' sealant.

Mouthguards

Almost 20% of British 12-year-olds are believed to have sustained some form of traumatic injury to their upper permanent incisors. In many cases,

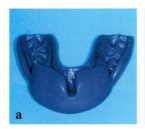 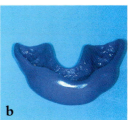

Fig 3-16 Custom-made mouthguards for sports showing (a) good and (b) poor extension into the labial sulcus.

the trauma may have been unavoidable, but sports-related injuries are largely preventable.

It should be recognised that children with an increased overjet, incompetent lips or with a past history of trauma are on a collision course for further trauma.

Any child that is involved in a contact sport (football, hockey, rugby, martial arts, and possibly cycling or horse-riding) should be provided with a custom-made sports guard (Fig 3-16a, b). The success of mouthguards in reducing dento-alveolar and even brain injury from an impact is undisputed. It is imperative, however, that the mouthguard extends sufficiently into the anterior labial sulcus, otherwise an impact can be directed on to the teeth themselves. It is also advisable to ask the technician to 'block off' any newly erupting teeth on the working model so that the guard will fit for a longer period of time. It is likely that a mouthguard will need to replaced annually in the growing child.

Mouthguards may also be considered for:
- children with uncontrolled epilepsy
- children with severe motor disabilities (who are more prone to trauma)
- patients with excessive tooth wear from attrition/erosion
- children with temporomandibular joint dysfunction
- patients suffering from oral trauma due to self-harm.

Practical Prevention: Putting it all Together

Some working examples of suggested preventive strategies for a number of different clinical scenarios are set out in Table 3-6.

Table 3-6 **Working examples of individualised preventive programmes**

Clinical Scenario	Suggested Preventive Programme
A two-year-old girl, living in a non-fluoridated region, presents with early cervical lesions on upper primary incisors. Her older sister required multiple extractions at five years of age	• show parent/s the lesions, explain the aetiology and explain what will happen if they progress • carry out a full dietary history, enquiring specifically about drinking habits (bottles at night) or prolonged breast-feeding. • recommend water or milk in feeder cups and advise against sugar-containing drinks at night • advise parents how to brush child's teeth using a children's toothpaste and recommend they rub additional paste onto the early lesions • apply fluoride varnish at three-month recall visits • consider fluoride supplements (tablets) at the age of three • regular recall
A five-year-old boy presents with stained occlusal fissures on all second primary molars. He has just started receiving fluoridated milk at school	• show parent/s the stained teeth, explain the aetiology and say what will happen if they progress • carry out a full dietary history, enquiring specifically about drinking habits and between-meal snacks. Suggest alternative 'safe' snacks. Watch out for hidden sugars in flavoured crisps and yoghurts, which may be perceived as 'good' snacks by the family • recommend that the mother supervises tooth brushing – using a children's toothpaste - to clean posterior surfaces well at least once a day • take bitewing radiographs to determine the extent of the caries. If limited to enamel, consider placing clear fissure sealants on occlusal surfaces and keep under regular radiographic review
A seven-year-old boy presents with a history	• reinforce dietary advice • disclose and check the boy's tooth-

Clinical Scenario	Suggested Preventive Programme
of a dental general anaesthetic for extraction of all primary molars at the age of four, but currently has no obvious caries	brushing technique • advise adult-dose fluoridated toothpaste • fissure-seal all erupted first permanent molars • regular recall
A 13-year-old boy, who is a keen footballer, presents with exposed dentine on the palatal surface of his upper permanent incisors but has no caries	• enquire about drinking habits, in particular sports drinks – advise water, or an occasional soft drink, through a straw • advise not to brush teeth after intake of carbonated drinks – rinse with water • if patient complains of sensitivity, apply fluoride varnish to eroded surfaces and recommend a desensitising fluoridated toothpaste • advise a daily 0.05% fluoride rinse (alcohol-free) to encourage remineralisation • consider fissure-sealing palatal surfaces if drink habit is likely to continue or moderate amounts of exposed dentine are present • ensure the patient is provided with a custom-made mouthguard for football • monitor degree of tooth tissue loss regularly (using study models and photographs)

Recommended Reading

British Society of Paediatric Dentistry. A policy document on fluoride dietary supplements and fluoride toothpastes for children. International Journal of Paediatric Dentistry 1996;6:139-142.

British Society of Paediatric Dentistry. A policy document on fissure sealants in paediatric dentistry. International Journal of Paediatric Dentistry 2000;10:174-177.

Clerehugh V, Tugnait A, Chapple I. Periodontal Management of Children, Adolescents and Young Adults. London: Quintessence, 2004.

Davis RM. The prevention of dental caries and periodontal disease from the cradle to the grave: what is the best available evidence? Dental Update 2003;30:170–179.

Ketley CE, West LJ, Lennon MA. The use of school milk as a vehicle for fluoride in Knowsley, UK; an evaluation of effectiveness. Community Dental Health 2003;20:83–88.
Levine RS, Stillman-Lowe CR. The scientific basis of oral health education. Lowestoft. British Dental Journal Books, 2004.

Ripa LW. Sealants revisited: an update of the effectiveness of pit and fissure sealants. Caries Research 1993;27(suppl):77–82.

Twetman S. Antimicrobials in future caries control? A review with special reference to chlorhexidine treatment. Caries Research 2004;38:223–229.

UK Clinical Guidelines in Paediatric Dentistry. Prevention of dental caries in children. International Journal of Paediatric Dentistry 1997;7:268–272.

Chapter 4
The Restorative Phase of Treatment

Aim

This chapter will provide an overview of the numerous restorative options that can be considered for the young dental patient.

Outcome

On reading this section, the practitioner will have gained an understanding of the most appropriate restorative approach to take in a wide range of clinical situations. In particular, the reader will have gained knowledge of:
- planning the sequence of restorative care
- selection of restorative materials
- management of pulpally involved teeth
- use of fixed and removable prostheses
- bleaching techniques.

Introduction

Why Bother Filling Primary Teeth?
Many practitioners do not routinely restore carious primary teeth. Opinions range widely as to whether this constitutes neglect or whether this may be a justifiable approach in some situations. Whichever approach is taken, the decision to restore or not to restore should always be based on a sound assessment of numerous factors including:
- age of the patient
- patient compliance and attendance pattern
- medical status
- caries risk
- rate of caries progression
- location and extent of caries
- presence/absence of the permanent successor.

For instance, a non–restorative approach may be indicated for:
- arrested or potentially arrestable caries (Fig 4-1)
- asymptomatic carious primary teeth that are close to exfoliation

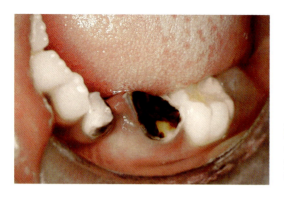

Fig 4-1 Arrested caries in second primary molar of a seven-year-old where a non-restorative approach is appropriate.

- extremely young or uncooperative patients who need further acclimatisation prior to attempting restorative treatments.

In cases where a decision is made not to restore carious primary teeth, the practitioner has a duty to review these teeth regularly, both clinically and radiographically, and to ensure that a rigorous preventive programme is in place.

On the other hand, arguments for filling carious primary teeth are as follows:
- to reduce the risk of an acute problem that may necessitate emergency treatment, including a general anaesthetic
- to avoid the need for more complex treatment, such as pulpotomies or extractions, should the caries progress
- to maintain the dental arch, thus reducing future orthodontic problems arising from space loss
- to help develop a positive attitude towards dental health in the child and the parent
- to acclimatise the child to accepting future dental treatment.

Where Does Restorative Treatment Fit into an Overall Treatment Plan?
Ideally, restorative intervention should start once:
- appropriate investigations have been undertaken
- any acute problems have been addressed
- a thorough preventive regime has been established
- patient cooperation is assured
- a specialist opinion has been sought in more complex cases.

There will always be patients who present with symptoms at their first visit. In such situations 'emergency' treatment will first be needed to relieve pain

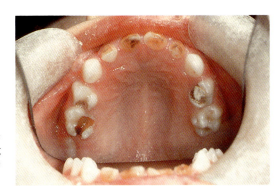

Fig 4-2 Extensive caries in the primary dentition requiring preventive and restorative intervention.

or infection before implementing the preferred treatment approach – prevention and acclimatisation first, intervention second. Furthermore, some patients may require a specialist Orthodontic, Restorative or Paediatric Dentistry opinion before starting an extensive course of treatment to ensure that longer-term treatment options are not compromised.

Sequence of Restorative Treatment

Suggestions for planning the restorative phase of treatment are as follows:
- Restore posterior teeth before anterior teeth. Once dental appearance has been improved, patients often fail to return for remaining posterior fillings.
- Given the choice, restore maxillary teeth before mandibular ones, as an infiltration is more acceptable to patients than inferior dental block anaesthesia.
- Plan to do simple quick restorations first, thus building the patient's confidence before undertaking more demanding work.
- Right-handed operators should start with a right quadrant and left-handed operators should start with the patient's left side to facilitate local anaesthetic administration.
- Try to limit the number of visits by doing 'quadrant' dentistry.

The Rampant Caries Case

One of the most difficult cases to plan and treat is the child with rampant caries (Fig 4-2). It is important to keep things in perspective and observe the following guidelines:
- Deal with any pain first.
- Instigate a rigorous preventive programme.
- Consider referral to a Paediatric Dentistry specialist if necessary.
- Identify key teeth that need to be retained and restored.

- Start a carefully planned sequence of restorations.
- Consider extraction of teeth of poorest prognosis.
- Limit the number of appointments by carrying out quadrant dentistry.
- If patient or parent compliance is being lost, it may be necessary for the patient (and operator) to have a break from the planned course of treatment.
- It may be necessary to further revise the treatment plan, depending on symptoms, the prognosis of various teeth and patient compliance.

With the primary dentition, treatment may be further complicated by a young and uncooperative child. Under such circumstances it may be preferable to simply try to stabilise disease progression by any of the following approaches:
- Use interdental polishing strips to clear contacts in primary incisors with interstitial caries, then regularly apply a fluoridated varnish.
- Place clear fissure sealants over early occlusal caries in primary molars until cooperation is assured. In the meantime, keep the teeth under close clinical and radiographic review.
- Use an excavator or large round bur in a slow handpiece (without local anaesthetic) to remove infected soft caries and place a glass–ionomer restoration, an approach known as the atraumatic restorative technique (ART).
- Undertake chemomechanical caries removal, using an agent such as Carisolv (a gel mixture of amino acids and sodium hypochlorite) and special hand instruments, to gradually remove infected dentine without the need for local anaesthetic or a handpiece, then restore with an adhesive material.

Where there are a number of primary teeth of poor prognosis, holding on to primary canines and second molars should be the priority, although parents are usually keener to maintain the incisors. In cases in which child and parental compliance is poor, and there are numerous teeth of poor prognosis, extractions under general anaesthesia may be the preferred approach. Indeed, this may be a kinder and more realistic approach than attempting to perform multiple pulpotomies followed by preformed crowns.

Matters are complicated in the secondary dentition, as extraction of permanent teeth is an option not to be taken lightly. When faced with caries in practically every tooth surface, it may be prudent to 'temporise' before placing definitive restorations (Fig 4-3a, b). The aim is to remove all caries and place zinc oxide eugenol dressings or 'temporary' glass ionomer restorations. The prognosis of each tooth can then be ascertained, and a more definitive treatment plan can be devised, possibly to include any endodontic treatment

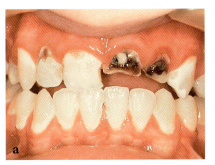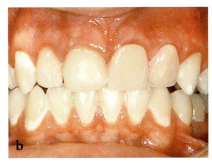

Fig 4-3 (a) Rampant caries in the permanent dentition: the primary aim is to stabilise disease progression before (b) comprehensive restorative input.

and extractions. Also, by this stage, the patient's attendance, attitudes and behaviour are better understood as factors to consider in planning longer-term treatment. The rampant caries case is not usually a candidate for orthodontic treatment. However, before embarking on endodontic therapy or permanent extractions an orthodontic assessment may be appropriate.

Use of Local Anaesthetic for Restorative Treatment

This is a controversial area in the management of the child patient. Why are some practitioners so reluctant to give children an injection before a filling? Is it fear of hurting the child, a means of saving time or a belief that children and their teeth are somehow less likely to feel pain than adults? The following points support the routine use of local analgesia when restoring children's teeth:

- Children are not decerebrate beings, so the use of local anaesthetic is strongly advocated for the majority of restorations.
- Inflicting pain while preparing a cavity in an unanaesthetised tooth is likely to create more patient management problems than would result from giving a careful injection in the first instance (Table 4-1).
- There is evidence that the use of local anaesthetic for restorative treatment correlates positively with the longevity of the restoration.

There may be some occasions, however, when a local anaesthetic is not indicated:

- temporisation of teeth with advanced physiological root resorption, as considerable intrapulpal neural degeneration will have occurred
- as part of a gradual acclimatisation process in very young or anxious children when only hand instruments or a slow handpiece can be used for caries removal

Table 4-1 **Tips for giving a successful local anaesthetic to children**

1.	**Prepare child for what is going to happen**	Depending on age and past experience, let the child know what you are going to do, using child-friendly and positive terminology – for instance: *for a very young child:* 'I'm just going to put your tooth to sleep with some special magic medicine' 'You have to be very still or the magic won't work' 'Your lip will feel a bit funny afterwards – like a jelly!' *for an older child:* 'I'm just going to squirt a little bit of sleeping medicine next to your tooth' 'You might feel a tiny scratch, or you might not feel anything at all' 'It tastes a bit nasty so we will get you a drink of water ready for straight afterwards'.
2.	**Prepare your equipment**	Ensure the local anaesthetic syringe is already loaded and out of sight – you don't want to alarm the child by furtive goings-on behind his or her back.
3.	**Apply lots of topical anaesthetic**	Topical anaesthetic is fantastic, and comes in nice flavours - a favourite being bubble gum. Apply it to dry mucosa on a cotton wool roll for about two minutes. When giving an inferior alveolar block, place the topical anaesthetic in a concavity made at one end of the cotton roll and apply between the pillar of fauces, and get the child to bite on the roll for a couple of minutes. Tell the child, that the 'jelly' might make the mouth feel a bit warm and tingly.
4.	**Distraction**	The art of a good local anaesthetic tech-

nique lies in distraction. Various techniques can be employed, depending on the child's age and past experiences of dental injections – for example:

for very young children:
talk constantly, tell them a story, tell them how good they are being, tell them to wiggle their toes or the magic won't work, ask them if they can hear their tooth snoring yet

for older children:
ask them to give you marks out of 10 depending on whether they felt anything or not (10 = felt nothing), chat while giving the local anaesthetic.

5.	**Local anaesthetic technique**	We can't really cover all the different techniques employed but suggest the injection is given slowly, into taut mucosa, with lots of accompanying chat. Intraligamentary injections can be a good alternative to a block, but they can sting – so giving a 'pain-free' buccal infiltration first is a good idea. Also, always use trans-papillary injections (following a buccal infiltration) as an alternative to a palatal injection, which usually hurts.
6.	**Avoid nasty tastes**	Children dislike the bitter taste of local anaesthetic solution, so keep a salivary ejector next to your syringe during administration of the local anaesthetic and have some water ready for rinsing immediately after the injection.
7.	**Post-op warnings**	Always remember to warn children and parents about inadvertent biting of anaesthetised tissues and the feeling of pins and needles as sensation returns.

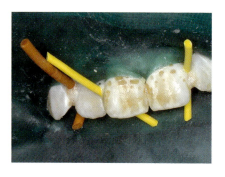

Fig 4-4 Rubber dam held in place with rubber 'wedjets' avoids the need for a clamp.

- when only chemomechanical caries removal is being undertaken
- for minimal preparation techniques, including air abrasion
- for minimal restorations in patients with a medical condition that may complicate local anaesthesia (in such cases inhalation sedation may be helpful).

Any treatment plan should include appropriate preparation of a child to accept local anaesthesia if it is required. Clinicians should also be aware of new techniques, such as computerised local anaesthesia (the 'Wand' system), which may be found to be acceptable to anxious children requiring local analgesia.

Use of Rubber Dam for Restorative Treatment

Most children are very happy to accept rubber dam, if it is appropriately introduced. It can be quick and easy to apply, in particular if dry dam and latex cord (wedjets) are employed (Fig 4-4). Rubber dam is strongly recommended in the following situations:

- endodontic treatment, to protect the airway and to isolate the oral tissues from potentially irritant medicaments
- in deep-cavity preparation to avoid the risk of bacterial contamination in cases in which pulpal exposure is a possibility
- for composite restorations when moisture control is critical
- to optimise cross-infection control in certain patients, including those with tuberculosis and HIV
- bleaching techniques, including microabrasion, to protect the oral tissues from inadvertent exposure to acid etchants and bleaching agents.

Restorative Materials

A number of restorative materials have a place in Paediatric Dentistry. In the primary dentition, patient cooperation and expected time until tooth exfoliation are the two main factors governing material selection. The decision-making process when choosing a restorative material for primary teeth is summarised in Fig 4-5.

Temporary Dressings

Temporary dressing selection is often a matter of personal preference and may include intermediate restorative material (IRM), polycarboxylate cement, zinc oxide eugenol and glass-ionomer cements. It is worth bearing in mind that young children can be very upset by the 'stingy' taste of zinc oxide eugenol.

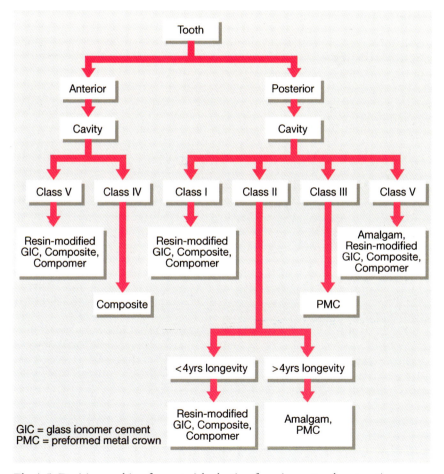

Fig 4-5 Decision-making for material selection for primary tooth restoration.

Glass–Ionomers

Conventional hand-mixed powder and water glass-ionomers have limited application as a restorative material, given their poor wear and strength characteristics.

Clinical applications

Glass-ionomer cements:
- as a luting cement for preformed metal crowns
- as a temporary dressing.

Resin-modified glass-ionomers, in contrast, are proving very popular in paediatric dental practice. These materials have favourable aesthetics, setting properties and wear characteristics. A number of studies have reported excellent three-year survival rates when the resin-modified glass-ionomers are used in Class I and II cavities in primary molars. The fluoride-containing characteristics of these materials may be of importance in the remineralisation process.

Clinical applications

Resin-modified glass-ionomers:
- in Class I and II primary molar cavities where the life expectancy of the tooth is less than four years
- in Class V cavities in primary and permanent teeth
- as an 'interim' restoration when trying to stabilise rampant caries cases or before placement of a more definitive restoration, such as a preformed metal crown
- in the atraumatic restorative technique or following chemomechanical caries removal
- as a base material in deep-cavity preparations.

Compomers

Compomers are polyacid-modified resins with similar applications to those of glass ionomer cements. The need for acid-etching and bonding, however, demands increased operator time and good patient compliance. Compomers have been shown to be as durable as amalgam restorations over a three-year period when used in aproximal primary molar cavities.

Clinical applications

Compomers:
- in Class I and II primary molar cavities where the life expectancy of the tooth is less than four years

- in Class V cavities in primary or permanent teeth
- as an interim restoration, before preformed metal crown placement.

Composites

Composites have excellent aesthetics, ease of use and reparability, making them invaluable and versatile restorative materials. Furthermore, their placement demands little sound tooth tissue destruction, which is of paramount importance in the young mouth. It is also worth mentioning flowable composites. This tooth-coloured, but 'runny' form of composite is extremely useful for temporary dentine coverage in fractured or eroded teeth.

Clinical applications

Composites:
- repair of fractured incisors with or without the use of celluloid crown forms
- labial and palatal restorations in eroded incisors
- restoration of carious anterior teeth with or without the use of celluloid crown forms
- preventive resin restorations in posterior teeth
- small occlusal restorations in posterior teeth
- as indirect and direct veneers in anterior teeth with enamel defects, such as amelogenesis imperfecta
- for altering tooth shape in, for example, the management of a microdont lateral incisor or 'conversion' of a canine to a lateral incisor
- as a splint for traumatised incisors with or without archwire
- for restoring infraoccluded primary molars to maintain vertical and antero-posterior space.

It is worth stating that pins should never be used in young patients due to the prominence of pulpal horns and the availability of excellent adhesive materials.

Amalgam

Does amalgam still have a part to play in the restoration of primary teeth? Its use in primary teeth has been discontinued in much of Scandinavia. In contrast, British Society of Paediatric Dentistry clinical guidelines state that amalgam can be used in primary teeth if it is considered the most appropriate material. Amalgams still outperform adhesive restorations in terms of longevity, but with the continued improvement of adhesive materials there are increasingly fewer indications for the use of amalgam in the primary dentition. Furthermore, the increased use of preformed metal crowns in the management of grossly carious primary molars obviates the need for multisurface amalgam restorations.

Clinical applications
Amalgams:
- single and multisurface cavities in posterior permanent teeth
- large Class II primary molar cavities when the life expectancy of the tooth is greater than four years
- polishing of amalgams is not recommended.

Preformed Metal Crowns
Preformed metal crowns (PMCs), traditionally known as stainless steel crowns are easy to use and highly durable, lasting much longer than a multisurface amalgam restoration in a primary molar (Fig 4-6a, b). Indeed, PMCs may be quicker to place (and thus more cost-effective) than a multisurface amalgam, which requires matrix band placement, packing and contouring. PMCs also have the added benefit of protecting all tooth surfaces against future caries attack. Cementation can be achieved either with a glass-ionomer or a polycarboxylate cement.

Tip: Before PMC placement on first permanent molars consider placing separators to open the contacts. The space created may well obviate the need for any tooth preparation. If possible, delay placement until the adjacent second primary molar has exfoliated so that only minimal (or no) tooth preparation is required.

Clinical applications
Preformed metal crowns:
- pulpotomised primary teeth that are brittle and subject to fracture
- in the management of large multisurface carious cavities in primary molars
- hypoplastic or grossly carious first permanent molars (in such situations the crown may be acting simply as an 'interim' restoration before tooth extraction or placement of a laboratory-formed crown)
- primary or permanent molars affected by abnormalities of tooth structure, including amelogenesis imperfecta or dentinogenesis imperfecta
- severely eroded primary or permanent posterior teeth
- as a fixed-space maintainer (with attached loop)
- to restore infraoccluded teeth to maintain vertical and horizontal space.

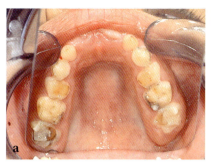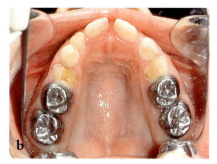

Fig 4-6 (a) Carious and eroded mixed dentition. (b) Restored with PMCs on upper second primary molars and first permanent molars.

Fixed Prostheses

There are limited applications for laboratory-made fixed prostheses in Paediatric Dentistry. It is better to delay the provision of crowns, bridges, veneers and implants until:

- growth has been completed
- gingival maturity has been achieved
- patients are able to care for such restorations.

Nonetheless, there are some situations were where fixed prostheses are indicated for the under-16s. These are considered below.

Porcelain Veneers

Porcelain veneers have an important part to play in improving the aesthetics of unsightly anterior teeth. Placement is usually delayed until patients reach their mid-teens (Figs 4-7 and 4-8).

Clinical applications

Porcelain veneers:

- to improve the shape of anterior teeth, such as microdont lateral incisors
- restoration of teeth affected by enamel defects (hypoplasias or opacities) when bleaching and composite restorations have not produced acceptable aesthetics
- restoration of incisors with extensive tooth tissue loss attributable to erosion
- repair of extensively fractured incisors.

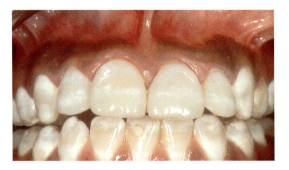

Fig 4-7 Porcelain veneers on upper central and lateral incisors with inclusion of 'enamel opacities' to match natural dentition.

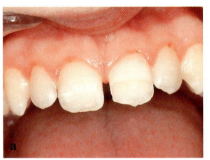

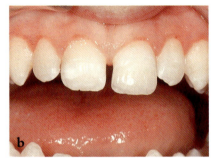

Fig 4-8 (a) Localised enamel hypoplasia affecting the incisal half of the upper left central incisor. (b) Restored with a partial (half tooth) porcelain veneer.

Tip: It can be quite a challenge to restore a single anterior tooth when the remaining dentition displays generalised enamel opacities, as might be seen in dental fluorosis or inherited enamel defects. Ensure that a good-quality photograph is sent to the technician so that dentine opaquers can be incorporated within the porcelain veneer to allow it to blend in with the natural teeth (Fig 4-7).

Full labial coverage is not always necessary. In Fig 4-8 only the incisal half of the upper central incisor is hypoplastic, the cervical region being normal. Thus a 'conservative' partial veneer was made. This avoided the need for any tooth preparation at the cervical margin.

Indirect Composite Restoration

Indirect composite restorations have a number of advantages over porcelain laminate veneers in the young patient:

- they are less costly
- they are easier to replace
- they can be readily modified/repaired
- it is relatively easy to bond an orthodontic bracket to a composite veneer.

Indirect composites can be made at the chairside (on a superglue-sealed stone model) or in the laboratory. There are a number of indications for their use.

Clinical applications
Indirect composite restorations:

- restoration of multiple hypoplastic teeth (particularly premolars), to save chairside time
- occlusal restoration of infraoccluded primary molars to maintain horizontal and vertical space
- management of severely discoloured teeth, with scope to use opaque/multiple shades.

Porcelain Crowns

These have very little, if any, part to play in the restoration of the young dentition, as extensive tooth tissue removal is required for such crowns.

Post Crowns

The use of post crowns is inappropriate in the management of the young dentition. In cases in which an anterior root has been retained, it is preferable to place a partial denture or an adhesive bridge over the root. Children are often prone to repeat trauma. Furthermore, the reduced dentine thickness seen in immature roots is not conducive to supporting a post crown and may result in vertical root fracture.

Metal Onlays

One may consider placing gold onlays on hypoplastic or eroded permanent molars in younger patients as an alternative to 'semi-permanent' preformed metal crowns (Fig 4-9a, b). Such onlays require minimal tooth preparation and, subject to technique, practically no occlusal adjustment after cementation. However, with continued developments in composites there are diminishing indications for the use of metal onlays.

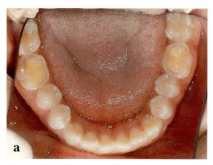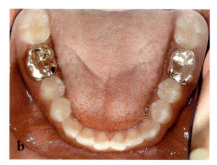

Fig 4-9 (a) Erosion of lower first permanent molars in a 12-year-old boy. (b) Restored with gold onlays.

Clinical applications
Metal onlays:
• certain hypoplastic or eroded permanent molars.

Adhesive Bridges
Although adhesive bridges have the disadvantage of a relatively high rate of cement failure, they have the considerable advantage of being minimally invasive to tooth tissue. Furthermore, if failure occurs, it is not catastrophic, as is usually the case with a failed post crown. Adhesive bridges are therefore indicated in Paediatric Dentistry for the replacement of missing anterior and premolar units.

Clinical applications
Adhesive bridges:
• replacement of an anterior tooth, lost due to trauma sequelae, caries or a dental anomaly
• interim replacement of an anterior crown, when the root is being retained until more definitive treatment (such as an implant) can be undertaken
• hypodontia cases, when multiple bridges are sometimes required.

Implants
Implants may be employed to replace missing teeth but are not usually considered until growth has been completed. There is growing interest in the use of implants to provide anchorage for tooth movement in selected orthodontic cases.

Removable Prostheses

Partial Acrylic Dentures

Partial acrylic dentures play a major role in Paediatric Dentistry - in particular, for the replacement of one or more missing permanent incisors. They are generally very well accepted by children and provide a good restorative option for the developing dentition.

Clinical applications

Partial acrylic dentures:

- replacement of an anterior crown when the tooth has suffered a cervical crown/root fracture
- replacement of an anterior tooth, lost due to caries or trauma sequelae
- replacement of an anterior tooth removed as a result of a dental anomaly (crown/root dilaceration, double tooth) or aberrant position
- replacement of congenitally missing teeth
- space maintenance, when the tooth has failed to erupt (and is awaiting surgical exposure) or when teeth are infraoccluded (submerged).

The preferred design for anterior tooth replacement is the 'T-shaped' acrylic denture (Figs 4-10, 4-11). Essentially, the denture margins are kept clear of the majority of teeth, thus limiting the development of marginal gingivitis and cervical caries. Furthermore, in the developing dentition posterior teeth can exfoliate or erupt, unhindered by the baseplate.

Tip: Where there is repeated fracture of the acrylic tooth from the denture, consider the inclusion of an anterior bite plane.

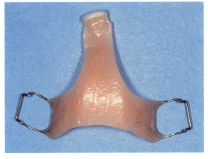

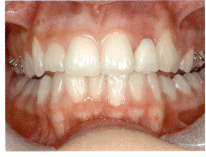

Fig 4-10 The 'T-shaped' acrylic denture: the ideal replacement for missing anterior teeth in children.

Fig 4-11 Temporary replacement of avulsed upper left lateral incisor with a 'T-shaped' denture.

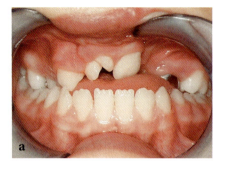

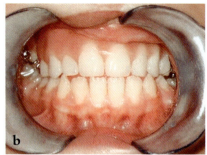

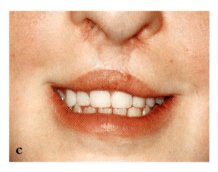

Fig 4-12 Use of an acrylic overdenture to improve aesthetics in a 13-year-old girl with bilateral cleft lip and palate(a) before treatment (b) and (c) with overdenture in place.

More conventional acrylic denture designs may be employed for patients with severe hypodontia. However, retention can be a problem in these patients given the conical nature of the teeth. This can be overcome by engaging cribs or clasps on preformed metal crowns or in conjunction with composite 'modification' to tooth shape.

Complete Acrylic Dentures/Overdentures
Provision of complete dentures or overdentures is sometimes indicated for patients with severe hypodontia. Overdentures may also be necessary for patients with cleft lip and palate when the maxillary segment is severely hypoplastic and there are numerous missing or malformed teeth (Fig 4-12).

Clinical applications
Full acrylic dentures or overdentures:
• severe hypodontia
• cleft lip and palate.

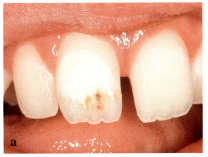 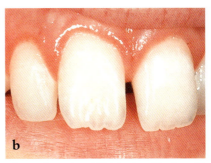

Fig 4-13 Removal of localised brown enamel opacity using 18% hydrochloric acid microabrasion technique (a) before treatment (b) after treatment.

Cobalt Chromium Dentures

Cobalt chromium dentures are not indicated in the developing dentition but are often employed in hypodontia patients, once growth is complete and the dentition has stabilised.

Bleaching

There are a number of clinical situations in which bleaching may be indicated in children. Some children may be subject to teasing at school as a consequence of the colour of their teeth. In selected cases, simple bleaching can greatly improve appearance. Indeed, bleaching may produce such a good cosmetic result that further, more invasive treatment is no longer required (Fig 4-13). Some of the indications for tooth-bleaching and the most appropriate treatment approach are summarised in Table 4-2.

Management of Pulpally Involved Teeth

Primary Dentition

A range of endodontic therapies can be employed in primary teeth and may be indicated for a variety of reasons, as shown in Table 4-3.

Pulpally compromised and non-vital anterior teeth are relatively easy to treat endodontically, although patient management can be difficult in the very young child. Pulpal contamination and necrosis may follow trauma, caries or extensive tooth tissue loss as a result of erosion. A preoperative periapical radiograph is essential and, if extensive periapical infection is noted,

Table 4-2 **Bleaching or tooth-whitening for children**

Clinical Indication	Approach	Comment
Dark, non-vital permanent anterior teeth that have been well obturated, have no associated periapical pathology and are not heavily restored	**'Walking bleach technique'** – hydrogen peroxide (30% solution) and sodium bicarbonate slurry is sealed within coronal pulp chamber for one to two weeks. Process is repeated until desired tooth colour is achieved	Ensure adequate gutta percha is removed, otherwise the tooth will remain dark at the cervical margin. To minimise subsequent cervical resorption, ensure a lining is placed over the radicular root filling to prevent diffusion of peroxide to the cervical periodontal ligament. Following bleaching, place a very light shade of composite restoration in the palatal access chamber
Vital teeth with unsightly demineralised (non-cavitated) lesions (possibly following orthodontic treatment)	**Microabrasion** – 18% hydrochloric acid and pumice slurry is very successful in removing post-orthodontic demineralised lesions, especially those that are a brown colour	Although considered a conservative technique, care must be taken not to remove too much tooth substance, otherwise the teeth will appear 'ditched' and yellow. Some operators advocate the use of 37% phosphoric acid gel, which is applied to the tooth surface using a rubber cup in a slow handpiece
Vital teeth with localised or generalised enamel opacities of white, yellow or brown colour that are of cosmetic concern to the patient	**Microabrasion** – (or the more conservative phosphoric acid and polish technique)	Microabrasion should be undertaken as the first line of treatment, even if composite or porcelain veneers are planned, to reduce any dark staining that may compromise future veneers

Table 4-3 **Indications and contraindications for pulp therapy in the primary dentition**

	Social Factors	Medical Factors	Dental Factors
Indications for pulp therapy	Well–motivated family, regular attenders Child or parent adverse to an extraction	Child has a bleeding disorder which would complicate an extraction	To maintain the dental arch To maintain the primary dentition in severe hypodontia cases To prevent development of aberrant oral habits following tooth loss
Contra-indications for pulp therapy	Poorly motivated family, irregular attenders (pulp-treated primary teeth must be kept under regular clinical and radiographic review	Child has a heart disorder putting him or her at risk of infective endo-carditis (potential for bacteraemia may remain from per-sisting chronic pulpal or intraradicular in-fection) Child is immuno-compromised (for example, oncology patient)	Tooth is unrestorable Tooth has less than two-thirds of root remaining Extensive soft- or hard-tissue infection Presence of internal pulpal resorption If contralateral tooth has already been re-moved it may be better to extract to prevent centre–line shift (for primary canines and first molars) Multiple grossly carious primary teeth (usually no more than two pulpotomies should be performed on a child)

extraction may be the preferred option. If endodontic treatment is indicated, pulpal extirpation (under rubber dam) should be followed by saline irrigation, gentle filing, drying with paper points and the placement of non-setting calcium hydroxide or pure zinc oxide eugenol paste in the pulp canal. The key consideration is to avoid any iatrogenic damage to the underlying permanent successor.

Extensively carious primary molars may frequently require pulp therapy. Studies have shown that, by the time marginal ridge breakdown has occurred, the coronal pulp is usually inflamed. Pulp therapy for primary molars, however, remains somewhat empirical, with paediatric dentists using a variety of different regimens. The table below (Table 4-4) outlines the most commonly accepted techniques and the rationale for their use. It should be noted that the use of formocresol in vital primary molar pulpotomy is now being superceded by the use of ferric sulphate, due to increasing concerns about the effect of formaldehyde. Practical details for undertaking primary pulp therapy and discussion regarding more novel approaches, such as the use of lasers, bone morphogenic proteins and mineral trioxide aggregate (MTA), can be found in some of the texts suggested for further reading.

One of the most important aspects of primary tooth pulp therapy is the follow-up – it is therefore not recommended for the irregular attender. It is important to review pulpotomised teeth clinically and radiographically to ensure that no pathological sequelae are occurring, such as radicular cyst formation (Fig 4-14). It is also important to ensure that the underlying successor continues to develop and erupt normally.

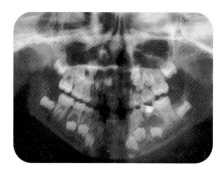

Fig 4-14 Radiographic evidence of radicular cyst formation in association with a pulpotomised lower left second primary molar.

Permanent Teeth

In child patients, success rates for direct pulp-capping (with hard-setting calcium hydroxide) are much better for permanent teeth than for the primary dentition. This is the recommended approach in cases of carious or traumatic pulp exposure, assuming the history is not suggestive of an irreversible pulpitis.

In cases of irreversible pulpits, pulpal extirpation is indicated. But before embarking on molar endodontics in a child, it should be ascertained as to whether it is in the child's best interests in the long term. Extraction may be the preferred option, especially if there is potential for physiological or orthodontic space closure. The status of the other first permanent molars should also be assessed carefully. Molar endodontics only tends to be indicated in:

- cases of severe hypodontia
- patients with bleeding disorders
- an intact well-aligned fully erupted permanent dentition in which only one tooth requires molar endodontics
- a well-motivated patient
- a tooth with mature apical development.

Endodontic procedures for traumatised permanent incisors will be discussed in Chapter five.

Special Restorative Problems

Table 4-5 highlights the more difficult and unusual restorative challenges that may be encountered in children. A brief summary is given for each, outlining a suggested management approach.

Recommended Reading

Bartlett D. Bleaching discoloured teeth. Dental Update 2001;28:14-18.

Beeley JA, Yip HK, Stevenson AG. Chemomechanical caries removal: a review of the techniques and latest developments. British Dental Journal 2000;188:427-430.

Deery C, Hosey MT, Waterhouse P. Paediatric Cariology. London: Quintessence, 2005.

Table 4-4 **Common pulpal therapies for primary molars**

Clinical Scenario	Technique	Comment
Grossly carious asymptomatic primary molar	Indirect pulp cap: remove soft caries avoiding pulp exposure, place calcium hydroxide or glass-ionomer cement lining	Good moisture control (rubber dam) and optimum coronal seal (adhesive restoration or preformed crown) are critical for a successful outcome (>90% success at 3-year follow up)
Traumatic pulp exposure during cavity preparation in an asymptomatic tooth	Direct pulp cap: arrest any pulpal bleeding and place calcium hydroxide lining over the exposure site	Good moisture control and optimum coronal seal are critical for a successful outcome. The approach is not recommended for carious pulpal exposures
Carious pulp exposure during cavity preparation in an asymptomatic vital tooth	Pulpotomy: remove entire coronal pulp and arrest radicular pulp bleeding using 15.5% ferric sulphate gel for 15 seconds, place zinc oxide eugenol or calcium hydroxide lining	This approach is increasingly being employed in preference to the formocresol pulpotomy due to concerns about the carcinogenic action of formaldehyde. It has good reported success rates (>90%) at 2-year follow-up
	N.B If coronal pulp proves too sensitive to remove, consider placement of a steroidal antibiotic paste (Ledermix™) directly over the pulp exposure for 7–10 days, before reattempting pulpotomy or pulpectomy procedure	

Clinical Scenario	Technique	Comment
Carious pulp exposure during cavity preparation in a vital tooth with clinical signs/symptoms of irreversible pulpal inflammation	One-stage pulpectomy: remove entire coronal and radicular pulp, carry out gentle filing, keeping 2mm short of apex. Irrigate with 0.5–1% sodium hypochlorite or chlorhexidine, dry and obturate canals with pure zinc oxide and eugenol or non-setting calcium hydroxide paste	Technically more demanding but theoretically the best approach with over an 80% success rate at 3-year follow-up
Infected non-vital tooth (likely to have an associated buccal sinus and/or radiographic radiolucency)	Two-stage pulpectomy: visit one as one-stage pulpectomy with calcium hydroxide paste sealed in canals for 1–2 weeks. Visit two – continue to latter stages of one-stage pulpectomy. If still frank infection, consider extraction.	

Table 4-5 **Special restorative challenges in children**

Condition	Management
Localised enamel defects	Consider pumice and etch technique or microabrasion first. May also require direct composite placement or porcelain veneer if opacity persists or tooth is hypoplastic.
Abnormal shape	Conical laterals can easily be restored with composite or porcelain veneers. Double teeth are a considerable problem, and a Paediatric Dentistry/Orthodontic opinion is advised before any restorative intervention. Ideally, any interventions should be delayed until apical closure has occurred, facilitating endodontic treatment, if this becomes necessary.
Erosion	Very little tooth preparation is required in cases of erosion. Restorations may be indicated to protect exposed dentine, alleviate sensitivity and improve aesthetics. Adhesive dentistry (including composites and cast metal onlays) and preformed metal crowns are invaluable approaches.
Generalised enamel defects	Consider specialist opinion in cases of severe generalised enamel defects such as amelogenesis imperfecta. The general principle is to place preformed metal crowns/onlays on posterior teeth and direct composites on anterior and premolar teeth. Consider definitive full occlusal coverage at 15–16 years of age.
Dentine defects	Same principles as for generalised enamel defects, but dentine defects are usually worse in the primary dentition, so treatment needs to start at a much earlier stage. Preformed metal crowns are invaluable and may be placed on all

Condition	Management
	primary molars. Strip crowns may be used for anterior primary teeth.
Infraoccluded primary teeth	If no successor, consider an orthodontic opinion as to whether it is beneficial to retain or extract. When teeth are to be retained, place a preformed metal crown, direct or indirect composite onlay, porcelain or gold crown to maintain space and function.
Cleft lip and palate	These patients should be under the care of a multidisciplinary team who will liase with the practitioner regarding restorative input. Patients commonly require composite modification of malformed anterior teeth and regrettably often suffer from a high caries experience.

Duggal MS, Curzon CEJ, Fayle SA, et al. Restorative techniques in paediatric dentistry. An illustrated guide to the restoration of extensively carious primary teeth. London: Martin Dunitz, 1995.

Forss H, Widström E. The post-amalgam era: a selection of materials and their longevity in the primary and young permanent dentitions. International Journal of Paediatric Dentistry 2003;13:158-164.

Hunter ML, Hunter B. Vital pulpotomy in the primary dentition: attitudes and practices of specialists in paediatric dentistry practicing in the UK. International Journal of Paediatric Dentistry 2003;13:246-250.

Ram D, Peretz B. Administering local anaesthesia to paediatric dental patients: current status and prospects for the future. International Journal of Paediatric Dentistry 2002;12:80-89.

Tinanoff N, Douglas JM. Clinical decision-making for caries management in primary teeth. Journal of Dental Education 2001; 65:1133-1142.

Chapter 5
Management of the Dental Emergency

Aim

This chapter will outline paediatric dental emergencies that commonly present in general practice. Appropriate management will be described briefly, but the main emphasis will be on the bigger picture - that is, how decision-making for emergency care should fit in with comprehensive treatment planning.

Outcome

On reading this section the practitioner should have a clear understanding of how to manage the following presenting problems:
- pain of pulpal origin
- orofacial infections
- trauma to the primary or permanent dentition
- non-accidental injury
- acute temporomandibular joint dysfunction
- oral lesions.

Introduction

Whose heart doesn't sink when informed that a patient in pain has just turned up at reception? With a busy schedule ahead, the 'problem' patient is exactly that, and more so if it is a child. Stress levels continue to rise if accompanying parents also become agitated. But bear in mind that parents may be anxious about dental treatment themselves or are at their wit's end after one or two sleepless nights, courtesy of their child's toothache. Dealing with the dental emergency is part of the job and can be extremely rewarding when the right approach is taken.

If the emergency patient is already in the middle of a course of treatment a decision has to be made as to whether the initial treatment plan now needs amending. If, however, the patient has presented for the first time, it is important to decide as to whether:
- only symptomatic primary treatment is indicated, as the patient is not likely to re-attend, or

- emergency care can be dictated by a longer term treatment plan, as the patient is going to attend for future care.

Principles of Management

The History

Good patient management starts with a good history. Taking a comprehensive patient history will help to ensure that the right diagnosis is reached and the most appropriate course of treatment prescribed. This is no less important when dealing with the emergency patient.

Children are not the most reliable historians, but it is worth asking a few key questions when trying to reach a diagnosis (Table 5-1). Obviously, the accompanying adult should be asked a number of questions, such as the time period over which the child has complained of pain, the use and effectiveness of any analgesics, details of recent dental treatment or trauma, episodes of swelling and whether symptoms are getting worse or better.

Examination and Special Investigations

Even in cases of a young or uncooperative child a careful examination should be undertaken. If the child fails to comply after initial gentle coaxing, he or she may need to be restrained in order to allow a thorough examination. This is a controversial area, and physical restraint should be undertaken only with parental consent. Furthermore, it is only appropriate for very young children and those with special behavioural problems that preclude them from complying. It is important to first explain to parents exactly what it proposed. Their active participation should be sought, and they should be reassured that their child will not be hurt in any way. It is best to lay the child across the mother's knee, with his or her head on the clinician's knee. The mother can hold the child's arms and the nurse restrain the legs, if necessary (Fig 5-1). A diagnosis and treatment plan should never be made in the absence of a proper examination.

- *Extraoral examination* – note whether the patient looks unwell or tired from lack of sleep. Is there any associated facial swelling or lymphadenopathy? If the child appears pyrexic, it is advisable to take the temperature (Fig 5-2), as a temperature >38°C may warrant hospital admission.
- *Intraoral examination* - look for caries, severe erosion, large or recent restorations, evidence of past trauma, and dental anomalies. Check if any teeth are mobile or tender (using only gentle finger pressure). Is there an

Table 5-1 **Key questions for a patient with reported toothache**

Question	Information Derived
1. Can you point at the tooth that hurts?	If the child is able to put a finger directly on a carious/heavily restored tooth it is likely that the tooth is non-vital and has an associated periapical infection or, more uncommonly, has a periodontal abscess
2. Does it hurt you at night?	If child has been kept awake an irreversible pulpitis is the most likely diagnosis
3. Has there been an associated extra- or intra-oral swelling?	If swelling is reported, the tooth is likely to be non-vital (or there may be a non–tooth-related swelling)
4. Is it painful when you bite on the tooth?	If yes, without history of disturbed sleep, the tooth is likely to be non-vital (or there may be a periodontal problem)
5. Do hot, cold or sweet things make the tooth hurt and, if so, for how long?	If pain occurs only on stimulus, in a permanent tooth, a reversible pulpitis is likely (or there may be exposed dentine from erosion, trauma or enamel hypoplasia). A diagnosis of reversible pulpitis is, however, more difficult to obtain for primary teeth, and in practice most are treated as if for an irreversible pulpitis

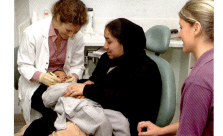

Fig 5-1 Young child being held to facilitate thorough dental examination.

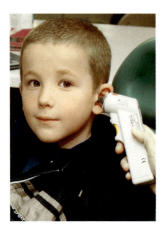

Fig 5-2 Taking an aural temperature.

associated sinus? Consider gentle periodontal probing if there is evidence of a periodontal problem.

- **Radiographs** – consider bitewings or lateral obliques for caries detection, periapicals if checking for intraradicular or periapical lesions, and an upper standard occlusal if trauma has been sustained to a number of maxillary incisors. A panoral radiograph may be indicated to check for the presence of all permanent successors and any dental or bony lesions.
- **Pulp sensibility** – pulp reactions to cold or electrical stimuli may be useful diagnostic aids but are probably best reserved for single-rooted permanent teeth in older (more reliable) children.
- **Other investigations** – it may be appropriate to consider further tests, such as a bacterial culture and sensitivity test (if there is frank pus exuding from an oral lesion), or baseline haematological or biochemical investigations, if an underlying systemic condition is suspected.

'Toothache'

The management of pain of pulpal origin is generally straightforward. If dealing with a primary tooth with spontaneous or prolonged pain, a pulpotomy/pulpectomy or extraction is indicated. The considerations for and against a pulpotomy have already been discussed (Table 3-2). When an extraction is planned it may be advisable to first relieve acute symptoms by carrying out a pulpotomy procedure and arranging for the extraction at a later stage. This may be undertaken when other phases of the treatment plan have been completed, cooperation is assured, or when alternative arrangements, such as referral for a general anaesthetic, have been made.

Analgesics including paracetamol (15mg/kg four-hourly) or non-steroidal anti-inflammatory drugs such as ibuprofen (5-10mg/kg eight-hourly) may be recommended for pain of pulpal origin. Antibiotics are not indicated in the absence of facial swelling or systemic symptoms.

Some key considerations when treatment planning for a child with an irreversible pulpitis are summarised in Table 5-2.

Table 5-2 **Treatment decisions for a patient presenting with irreversible pulpitis**

Primary Tooth	Permanent Tooth

• First take bitewing radiographs (or lateral obliques) to determine the overall caries experience, as this is one of the most important factors in treatment planning	• Is an extraction preferable to root treatment? Molar endodontics is a demanding procedure and may not be in the child's best interest. It is only indicated if:
	  1) the child has severe hypodontia, *or*
	  2) the child has a bleeding disorder that contraindicates surgery, *and*
	  3) the child is a very compliant and regular attender, *and*
	  4) the molar in question has mature apical development

• Is a pulpotomy indicated, or is it better to extract the tooth (see Table 3.2)?	
• If extraction becomes necessary, should balancing extractions be undertaken (for primary canines and first primary molars)?	Certainly, it is usually preferable to extract a first permanent molar with irreversible pulpitis in a young patient where the second permanent molars have not yet erupted (see Chapter 2)
• Following extraction of a second primary molar, a space maintainer may	• If extraction of a permanent molar is indicated, the status of the other molars should also be assessed. An orthodontic

Primary Tooth	Permanent Tooth
be used to prevent mesial drift of the first permanent molar – providing the patient is compliant, is at low risk of caries and a regular attender	opinion may be advisable before the extraction, to see if any other teeth should be removed at the same time
• If an extraction under general anaesthesia is indicated, it is recommended that any other teeth of poor prognosis are also extracted to avoid future problems or a repeat anaesthetic	

Referral for Extractions under General Anaesthesia

Following relief of acute symptoms, young and uncooperative children with multiple teeth of poor prognosis may require referral for extractions under general anaesthesia. Once this decision has been made, treatment should be carefully planned as follows:

• Try to complete all necessary restorations before the general anaesthetic, as it cannot be assumed that the patient will comply with treatment after the general anaesthetic. If the patient does not comply a second general anaesthetic may be necessary if unrestored carious teeth subsequently become symptomatic. In view of the risks associated with general anaesthesia and the preventable nature of dental disease, the primary aim should be to avoid the need for a repeat procedure.

• Request removal of all teeth of poor prognosis. A radical approach is usually indicated when treatment planning for general anaesthesia. All teeth of poor prognosis should be extracted to avoid the possibility of future problems.

• Assess the condition of the first permanent molars. If one first permanent molar is of very poor prognosis, the condition of the other first permanent molars should also be carefully assessed together with the patient's compliance and overall orthodontic status. It may be of long-term advantage to remove more than one first permanent molar at the most appropriate stage of dental development (as discussed in Chapter 2).

- Check for severe erosion or trauma involving upper primary incisors. Young children requiring extraction of grossly carious primary molars may also demonstrate erosion. It is therefore prudent to assess upper primary incisors for tooth tissue loss. If advanced erosion is present in a child under five or six years of age there is a risk that pulpal necrosis will ensue before the natural exfoliation of the tooth. It is therefore necessary to either restore eroded incisors before the general anaesthetic, or to request their removal along with the carious primary molars. In addition, upper primary incisors should be carefully examined for evidence of past trauma. Non-vital primary incisors may warrant extraction.

- Consider the need for balancing extractions for primary canines and first primary molars. In addition to preventing centre line shift, removal of a contralateral first primary molar has the added advantage of removing a potentially carious contact in children at high risk of caries.

- Provide full information to parents or guardians regarding the risks of general anaesthesia. It is the duty of the referring practitioner to discuss the alternatives to a general anaesthetic and the risks associated with general anaesthesia. This should be documented in the patient's records. It is best not to promise a general anaesthetic, as the person providing the service ultimately decides on the appropriateness of this approach.

- Be aware of local waiting times for the provision of out- or in-patient general anaesthesia. Where there are long waiting times, it may be necessary to provide interim care to reduce the likelihood of problems occurring while the patient is on a waiting list for specialist treatment.

Orofacial Infections

The most common orofacial infections likely to be encountered in children and the appropriate courses of action are highlighted in Table 5-3.

Bacterial Infections

Most acute, rapid-onset, facial swellings in children have a dental aetiology (Fig 5-3a, b). Sometimes, but not always, there is a history of toothache, trauma or recent dental treatment. Very occasionally, a patient may present with an acute swelling of the upper lip in the absence of caries, erosion or trauma. In such cases, there may be a dens-in-dente (Fig 5-4), as pulpal necrosis and ensuing cellulitis can sometimes occur before the tooth has fully erupted.

Table 5-3 **Common orofacial infections in children**

Infection	Key Presenting Features	Primary Management
Bacterial		
Periapical/intra-radicular abscess (in absence of facial swelling)	• tender ± mobile non-vital tooth • buccal (occasionally lingual) swelling or sinus	• start endodontic treatment or extract • analgesics if necessary
Facial cellulitis (of dental aetiology)	• diffuse, tender, warm swelling, overlying skin appears erythematous • pyrexia • submandibular lymphadenopathy • trismus	• antibiotics and analgesics • endodontic treatment/ extraction of non-vital tooth as soon as possible • hospital admission for surgical drainage and intravenous antibiotics may be necessary
Periodontal abscess	• yellowish or red, soft, painful swelling of the gingiva • pus may exude from the gingival margin • associated tooth may be tender and mobile	• try to achieve drainage via gingival crevice • if possible, irrigate pocket with chlorhexidine via blunt needle and syringe • antibiotics and analgesics
Pericoronitis	• enlarged, erythematous, ulcerated operculum overlying partially erupted tooth • pus often exuding from operculum • may be associated extra-oral swelling • pyrexia • submandibular lymphadenopathy • trismus	• if possible, irrigate under operculum with chlorhexidine via blunt needle and syringe • give oral hygiene instruction and advise regular warm saline/ chlorhexidine mouthwashes • antibiotics and analgesics

Infection	Key Presenting Features	Primary Management
Acute suppurative sialadenitis	• painful swelling, usually unilateral, involving parotid gland, but may involve submandibular or sublingual glands • associated duct may appear inflamed and purulent liquid released • pyrexia • submandibular lymphadenopathy • trismus	• antibiotics and analgesics • removal of sialolith (stone) if present, once acute infection resolved
Impetigo	• very contagious staphylococcal or streptococcal skin infection • frequently involves circumoral region • presents as small macules that coalesce and form yellow/brown crusted lesions	• refer child to general medical practitioner for appropriate treatment
Viral *Acute herpetic gingivostomatitis*	• see Table 3-4	• see Table 3-4
Herpangina	• acute pharyngitis • febrile illness • multiple herpes-like ulcers with erythematous halo involving soft palate and pharyngeal mucosa	• symptomatic support – fluids, bed rest • analgesics

Infection	Key Presenting Features	Primary Management
Hand-foot-and-mouth-disease	• very infectious, usually a history of local out-break • mild systemic upset • vesicular rash involving fingers, toes, buttocks and oral mucosa	• symptomatic support (condition is not usually painful)
Infectious mononucleosis	• sore throat • cervical lymphadenopathy • petechia/erythema of soft palate	• haematological and serological investigation to confirm diagnosis • symptomatic support
Mumps	• tender and oedematous swelling of one/both parotid glands, submandi-bular or sublingual glands occasionally involved • pyrexia • submandibular lymphadenopathy • trismus	• symptomatic support • analgesics
Fungal *Thrush (pseudomem-branous candidosis)*	• white/yellow plaques easily removed with gauze to reveal erythematous mucosa • primarily involves tongue, cheeks or palate • usually seen in neonates following contamination from mother or feeding bottles	• consider gram-stained direct smear to confirm diagnosis • Nystatin pastilles or oral suspension 100,000 units four times a day until resolution • failure to respond to anti-fungal treatment warrants further investigation

Infection	Key Presenting Features	Primary Management
Chronic erythematous candidosis	• erythematous area of mucosa limited to fitting surface of denture or removable appliance • asymptomatic	• consider gram–stained direct smear to confirm diagnosis • advise about denture wear and hygiene • Nystatin pastilles or oral suspension 100,000 units four times a day until resolution

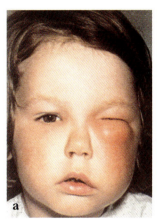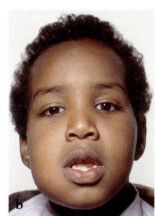

Fig 5-3 Typical presentation of facial cellulites in young children originating from a) non-vital maxillary tooth and b) non-vital mandibular tooth.

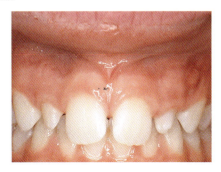

Fig 5-4 Chronic sinus associated with non-vital upper left permanent lateral incisor (dens-in-dente).

111

In cases in which the patient has a facial cellulitis secondary to pulpal necrosis, the primary aim is to remove the necrotic tissue and achieve drainage by pulpal extirpation or tooth extraction. In some instances the tooth may be too tender to touch and antibiotics are the first line of action. In such cases the following regimes should be followed:

- three gram sachet of amoxicillin followed by a further 3g eight hours later (half dose for children <10 years), or
- five-day course of amoxicillin, 250mg three times daily (half dose for children <10 years), or
- for children with a penicillin allergy, consider a 3-day course of metronidazole, 200mg three times daily (or 7.5mg/kg for young/small children).

When prescribing antibiotics for children it is important to:
- Enquire about previous experience of penicillin and any adverse reactions.
- Enquire about recent antibiotic use for other infections.
- Check whether tablets or a liquid preparation is more acceptable.
- Specify on the prescription that a sugar-free preparation is required.
- Give appropriate instructions and cautions for the antibiotic prescribed.

A point worth noting is that, for patients at risk of an infective endocarditis, it may be advisable to prescribe metronidazole in the first instance to reduce the acute infection. Amoxicillin can then be used as the prophylactic antibiotic of choice to cover a subsequent extraction. In severe infections, or in immunocompromised patients, a simultaneous course of amoxicillin and metronidazole should be prescribed. Regular paracetamol intake will help to keep the temperature down. The patient should be reviewed within 48 hours to ensure that the swelling is resolving and local measures should be instigated as soon as possible. An urgent hospital referral is warranted if:

- There is extensive extraoral swelling, with limited opening, or there is swelling involving the floor of the mouth which may compromise the airway.
- The patient is severely medically compromised.
- The child is listless and dehydrated (ask about urinary output).
- The child has a spiking pyrexia with temperatures over 38°C.
- The child is very young.

Antibiotics are not indicated for localised intraoral swellings in the absence of systemic upset, as such swellings can be managed locally. Over-prescription of antibiotics by the dental profession is reportedly a matter of growing concern.

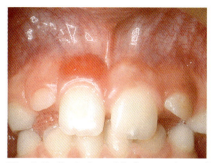

Fig 5-5 Periodontal inflammation of the upper right permanent central incisor caused by subgingival foreign body.

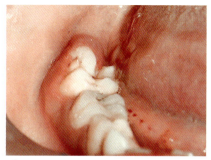

Fig 5-6 Pericoronitis involving a partially erupted lower first right permanent molar.

Periodontal abscesses are not common in children, but affected individuals may present with pain, in particular on biting, and localised swelling. The periodontal inflammation may be due to a foreign body, such as a fingernail being forced down the periodontal ligament (Fig 5-5). A lateral periodontal abscess may also occur as an acute manifestation of generalised periodontal disease, such as juvenile periodontitis. Occasionally children may present with facial swelling with or without trismus secondary to a pericoronitis. This is most commonly seen in association with partially erupted mandibular first or second permanent molars (Fig 5-6).

Non-odontogenic infections may also present with extraoral swelling. These may include soft tissue abscesses or salivary gland infections (acute suppurative sialadenitis).

Viral Infections
Acute herpetic gingivostomatitis is the most frequent acute viral infection to involve the oral mucosa and is not an uncommon 'emergency' presentation (see Table 3-4). A differential diagnosis for acute herpetic gingivostomatis may include herpangina, hand, foot and mouth disease, infectious mononucleosis, and varicella zoster virus.

Facial swellings of a viral aetiology are usually caused by mumps (epidemic parotitis). The parotid gland is normally involved, but occasionally the submandibular or sublingual glands are also affected. The reduced uptake of the MMR vaccine is likely to see an increase in the number of cases seen.

Fungal Infections

Thrush (pseudomembranous candidosis) may be seen in neonates as a white or yellow plaque involving the tongue, lips, cheeks or palate (see Table 3-4). It may also present in older children where there is reduced resistance to infection, an immunodeficiency, xerostomia, or following antibiotic therapy.

Trauma

Appropriate acute trauma management and subsequent treatment planning are critical in the young patient. Poor initial treatment may result in a prolonged course of treatment or the unnecessary loss of a tooth. This, in turn, has considerable economic, psychological, aesthetic and functional implications in adulthood. Furthermore, close post-trauma review is essential, ensuring that any loss of vitality, pathological changes, or disturbed development is diagnosed early. This will ensure that appropriate treatment is instigated sooner rather than later. Listed below are some key considerations when treatment planning for the child who has sustained dental trauma.

Stage of Dental Development

If trauma has occurred to primary incisors in a child under four years of age, the crown of the developing successor may have been damaged, in particular if the injury was an intrusion or avulsion (Fig 5-7). It is therefore important to be aware of possible sequelae such as enamel opacities, hypoplasia, dilacerations or arrested tooth development or eruption disturbances. The vitality and exfoliation of the traumatised primary tooth should be kept under close review, as should the eruption of the permanent successor (Fig 5-8).

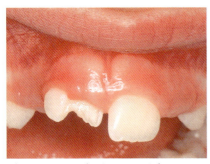 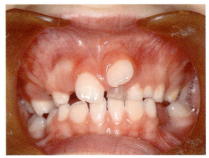

Fig 5-7 Hypoplastic upper right permanent central incisor following previous trauma to primary incisor.

Fig 5-8 Retained and discoloured upper left primary central incisor following trauma, with displacement of erupting successor.

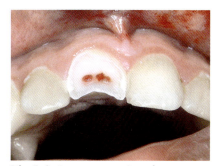

Fig 5-9 Large traumatic pulp exposure in immature central incisor, necessitating partial pulpotomy.

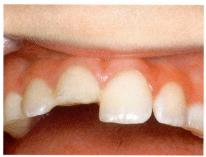

Fig 5-10 Composite 'bandage' for immediate dentinal coverage following uncomplicated crown fracture of the upper right permanent central incisor.

If trauma has occurred to primary incisors in a child over four years of age, sequelae may involve the root of the tooth, including dilacerations, arrested development, or displacement. Again close review of the injured primary tooth and permanent tooth eruption should be undertaken.

Where trauma has involved a permanent incisor, prognosis and treatment options may depend on the stage of dental development. For instance, avulsed or luxated (displaced) teeth with very immature apical development (open apices) will have a better chance of revascularisation and reinnveration than those with a fully mature apex. Thus monitoring tooth vitality in replanted immature teeth is justified, whereas pulp extirpation should be instigated for more mature teeth, which have no chance of revascularisation. Another development–related treatment decision relates to pulp exposures. In immature teeth with large pulp exposures (Fig 5-9), or even near exposures, it may be prudent to carry out an elective partial pulpotomy rather than pulpectomy. This entails the removal of contaminated coronal pulpal tissue and placement of calcium hydroxide powder and hard-setting calcium hydroxide lining over the remaining pulp. The primary objective is to maintain pulp vitality and continued root development, thus avoiding a prolonged course of treatment to achieve apical barrier formation using non-setting calcium hydroxide paste.

Delay in Treatment
Following trauma, any delay in treatment provision may adversely affect tooth prognosis. Replantation of an avulsed permanent incisor is usually expedited, but dentinal coverage of a fractured crown may not assume such

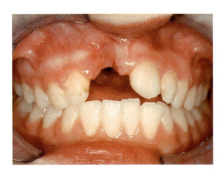

Fig 5-11 Extensive alveolar resoption following loss of the upper right permanent central incisor in a teenage girl.

high priority. A delay in covering exposed dentine may well result in pulpal contamination and resultant necrosis, which could have been avoided by early treatment. This does not mean that a definitive composite restoration need be placed on the day of the trauma. Hard setting calcium hydroxide and flowable composite (composite 'bandage') should, however, be placed over the exposed dentine, until definitive treatment can be carried out (Fig 5-10). The composite build-up should not be delayed for too long though, as opposing teeth may over-erupt or contralateral teeth may encroach on the space required for the definitive restoration.

Tip: When placing a temporary composite 'bandage' over sensitive, exposed dentine avoid the use of the 3-in-1 syringe. Instead use cotton pledgets moistened in warm water to remove the etchant. This is much more comfortable for the patient that a blast of cold water.

Patient Cooperation
In certain cases it may not be the best plan to replant an avulsed tooth, although this is a difficult decision to make. In children with a severe learning disability, and where the risk of repeat trauma is considerable, it may not be prudent to replant a tooth of poor prognosis, in particular if the child is unable to accept subsequent treatment in the dental chair.

Maintaining Roots and Alveolar Bone
Treatment planning for the young trauma patient should be mindful of keeping options open for the future. This is particularly pertinent when faced with, what seems, a hopeless situation following a crown/root fracture. In such instances, it is best to avoid extraction of the root, if at all possible, as considerable alveolar resorption may ensue (Fig 5-11). It is preferable to

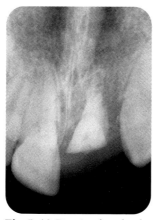

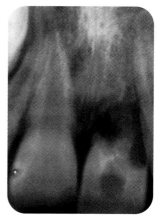

Fig 5-12 Retained and submerged upper left central incisor root to maintain alveolar bone.

Fig 5-13 Maintenance of alveolar bone despite continued replacement resorption of replanted upper left central permanent incisor.

retain the root either as a submerged vital root, if the fracture is below the margin of crestal bone (Fig 5-12) or as a non-vital root, if endodontic treatment is necessary. Maintaining the root and the supporting bone keeps options flexible for the future, facilitating provision of adhesive bridges, post crowns (with or without orthodontic extrusion or crown lengthening) or implant placement. Even where continued root resorption is taking place (Fig 5-13), roots can be left in situ if replacement bone is being laid down and there is no associated periapical infection.

Intermediate restoration of a lost crown is usually best achieved by means of a simple T-shaped acrylic denture (Figs 4-10 and 4-11). When the laboratory is pushed for time, a simple Essex retainer with or without an incorporated acrylic tooth provides an excellent, and easily constructed, space maintainer (Fig 5-14).

Orthodontic Considerations
Treatment planning, even for the acute trauma case, should include consideration of the patient's overall orthodontic status. As an example, Fig 5-15 shows how primary trauma management was carried out in conjunction with some simple orthodontic treatment. Some orthodontic factors to bear in mind when making treatment decisions for the trauma case are described below.

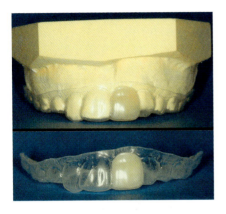

Fig 5-14 Essex retainer incorporating an acrylic tooth to provide a convenient and aesthetic 'emergency' space maintainer.

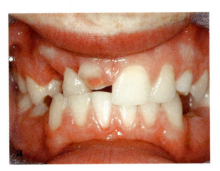

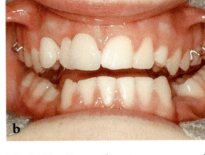

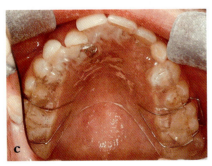

Fig 5-15 Comprehensive trauma and orthodontic treatment planning for a 13-year-old boy presenting with (a) an avulsed (and lost) upper right permanent canine and complicated crown fracture of the upper right central incisor who received (b) pulp extirpation and composite build-up of central incisor and (c) a removable orthodontic appliance to push the upper right lateral incisor over the bite, with an acrylic tooth to replace the upper right canine.

In patients with severe anterior crowding replantation of an avulsed tooth of poor prognosis may not be the best long-term solution. In a few cases it may be preferable to allow the eruption, and mesial drift, of a lateral incisor (which will bring new bone with it). Orthodontic and restorative intervention, as clinically indicated, can then be considered in the future.

In cases where the prognosis of a traumatised anterior tooth is very poor, it is worth considering the merit of autotransplantation of a single-rooted pre-molar to replace the anterior tooth. Obviously, an orthodontic opinion is advisable first, but in selected cases with posterior crowding, autotransplantation of a premolar tooth (ideally with no greater that 75% root development) may be a viable specialist treatment option.

Patients who have sustained trauma and are about to start orthodontic treatment, or who are in the middle of orthodontic treatment, need careful management. Following any trauma, the orthodontist should be contacted and advised of the incident. It is prudent to refrain from applying any forces to traumatised teeth for a short period of time after the impact, and to apply only light forces throughout the subsequent course of treatment. Another issue relates to endodontic therapy and orthodontic treatment: should non-vital teeth be root-filled before or after active tooth movement? It is prudent to maintain calcium hydroxide paste in the root canal until completion of orthodontic treatment, in particular if inflammatory root resportion is a possibility. In mature teeth that have not suffered damage to the periodontal ligament, obturation with gutta percha is not contraindicated prior to orthodontic treatment.

Medical Status
Patients who are at risk of infective endocarditis or who are severely immuno-compromised should be very carefully managed following dental trauma, in particular if endodontic treatment is required. It may be wise to refer such patients to a specialist.

Risk of Repeat Trauma
Patients who have sustained one episode of dental trauma are known to be at much greater risk of sustaining further dental trauma. This may be because they are just accident-prone, their teeth are already compromised from the initial trauma, or they are predisposed because of some dental factor (increased overjet), physical or medical disability (poor motor control, epilepsy) or participate in trauma-risk activities. Treatment planning for these patients should certainly include limiting the risk of future trauma by reducing overjet and/or providing custom-made mouthguards for sports.

Tooth Colour Changes
It is common to see colour changes in traumatised primary incisors. Typically, the crown appears a pink or grey colour shortly after the injury subsequent to pulpal haemorrhage (Fig 5-16). Quite often, a pink colour will

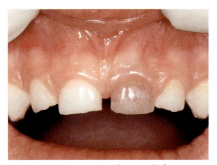 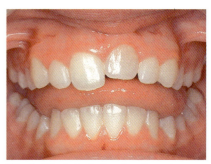

Fig 5-16 Traumatised upper left primary central incisor showing colour change but no associated periapical pathology.

Fig 5-17 Ankylosis of replanted upper left permanent central incisor.

resolve after a few weeks as pulpal blood products within the dentine tubules are resorbed. A yellow discolouration may be evident following pulp obliteration. Colour change alone, in the absence of any other signs and symptoms, is not an indication for intervention. The discoloured tooth should, however, be monitored clinically and radiographically for any signs of periapical infection. Appropriate action can then be taken.

Ankylosis

It is important to watch for signs of ankylosis in luxated and replaced avulsed teeth (Fig 5-17). Permanent anterior teeth that become infraoccluded ('submerged') and sound abnormal on percussion (giving a 'cracked tea-cup' sound) may create considerable cosmetic difficulties in the future. In some cases, it may be advisable to decoronate or extract these teeth rather than leave them to become severely infraoccluded with a distorted gingival contour. Non-vital primary teeth need to be monitored carefully to ensure that they exfoliate normally. If they do not, there is a risk of ectopic, or failed, eruption of the permanent successor.

Fractures of Facial Bones and Soft–Tissue Injury

Primary management of facial fractures and severe soft-tissue injury is likely to fall under the remit of the oral and maxillofacial surgeons (Fig 5-18). Such cases warrant urgent referral, in particular if the patient has sustained a head injury. The long-term follow up of such patients may, however, be the responsibility of the dental practitioner. It is thus important to be vigilant in monitoring for any disturbances to dental development or facial growth, with referral to a specialist centre as appropriate.

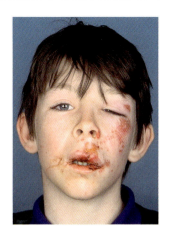

Fig 5-18 Eleven-year-old boy with severe abrasion injuries sustained by falling off a bicycle.

The dental practitioner may well be presented with minor soft-tissue injuries that need careful cleaning with saline and gauze. This facilitates the examination of the extent of the injury and usually makes things look much better. It is important to ensure that no foreign body is present in the wound and that the patient has had tetanus prophylaxis. Gaping extraoral wounds should be sutured and may warrant referral to a trauma unit or plastic surgeon. It is also important to ensure that displaced interdental papillae are repositioned and sutured. Lacerations to the tongue rarely need suturing, as healing occurs rapidly.

The main aim of this section has been to emphasise how trauma management should reflect long-term treatment objectives. The text could not describe the detailed management of every type of dental injury, but some broad guidelines are given in Table 5-4.

Non-Accidental Injury

It is important to be aware of signs of non-accidental injury (NAI) in young patients who present with repeated or unusual trauma. Typically NAI may present with:

- bruises that take the shape of a recognisable object and occur in odd places – not restricted to bony prominences
- injuries of different vintage
- a delayed presentation
- a history that is vague or inconsistent with the presenting injury
- a withdrawn, unhappy child.

Table 5-4 **Key points for dental trauma management**

Injury	Management
Primary tooth	*In all cases monitor the injured primary tooth (and adjacent teeth) clinically and radiographically for any loss of vitality, associated pathology or failure to exfoliate normally. Also monitor the development of permanent successors. Consideration for permanent successors should dictate treatment approaches for traumatised primary teeth*
Uncomplicated crown fracture	• fracture only into enamel – smooth, apply some Duraphat™ • fracture into dentine – apply calcium hydroxide lining and flowable composite just to cover dentine. If patient is very compliant you could restore fully with composite
Complicated crown fracture	• extraction is usually indicated. If very compliant patient (and desperately keen parents) could extirpate, fill root canal with non-setting calcium hydroxide paste, restore and monitor clinically and radiographically
Concussion, subluxation	• soft diet and analgesics, corsodyl on sponges
Luxation	• if the crown is displaced palatally, extract if in traumatic occlusion or very mobile, other wise leave to firm up – with supportive advice. Don't try to reposition, as doing so might damage the successor • if the crown is displaced labially, the root will be impinging on the permanent tooth, so try to reposition gently or extract • if extruded, leave if not in traumatic occlusion or excessively mobile – otherwise extract

Injury	Management
Intrusion	• leave tooth to re-erupt with supportive advice. If the tooth fails to re-erupt within two to three weeks, extraction may be necessary
Avulsion	• do not replant, as this will necessitate endodontic treatment of the avulsed tooth and may damage the successor. Advise parents about possible damage to successor, depending on age at which the trauma happened
Root fracture	• an unusual injury in primary teeth: leave under review unless the coronal portion is extremely mobile or becomes non-vital, in which case extract the coronal part but don't go digging for root, as this risks damage to successor.
Permanent tooth	*In all cases monitor the injured permanent tooth (and adjacent teeth) clinically and radiographically for any loss of vitality or associated pathology. Follow up for at least 2 years.*
Uncomplicated crown fracture	• fracture into enamel - smooth, apply some Duraphat™ varnish or dentine bond • fracture into dentine – place setting calcium hydroxide and composite bandage (definitive restoration may be carried out a few weeks later). If the patient has retained the fractured crown, consider bonding this to the remaining tooth
Complicated crown fracture	• if exposure very small and recent, consider pulp-capping and composite restoration

Injury	Management
	• if exposure is large in an immature tooth, consider partial pulpotomy ('Cvek technique'). If dealing with a mature tooth, extirpate
Concussion, subluxation	• soft diet and analgesics
Root fracture	• splinting for three months for a mid-root fracture • apical third fractures can usually be left unsplinted • if fracture is at cervical margin, remove crown, extirpate if fracture is above the level of crestal bone in a mature tooth or carry out pulpotomy in immature tooth • if facture line is below level of crestal bone, consider root burial by using a coronally repositioned flap over the root (don't take this approach if there is any periapical pathology present) • take impression for space maintainer
Luxations	• if the crown is displaced, and is mobile, reposition digitally or with forceps. Splint extrusive luxations for three weeks and lateral luxations for six to eight weeks • severe luxations in mature teeth will need extirpation after seven days
Intrusion	• if very immature tooth, and less than 6mm intrusion, could leave to re-erupt with supportive advice • in severely intruded immature tooth or intruded mature tooth, reposition using forceps or rapid orthodontic extrusion • endodontic treatment will need to be instigated in mature teeth after a couple of weeks

Injury	Management
Avulsion	• replant and splint for seven to 10 days • review splint at 48 hours • prescribe antibiotic course • if mature tooth, extirpate after a week • if immature tooth, keep under close review and extirpate if signs of inflammatory root resorption or periapical infection • if avulsed tooth was kept dry for a prolonged period, clean tooth, extirpate pulp, place in 2% NaF for 20 minutes and obturate extraorally before replanting and splinting for six weeks. The aim is to achieve ankylosis. This approach is therefore more appropriate in patients where growth is complete.

Concerns should be discussed immediately through the appropriate channels, which will vary according to each health authority. Practitioners should therefore familiarise themselves with correct local protocols for reporting suspected NAI before the event.

Acute Temporomandibular Joint Dysfunction

Acute temporomandibular joint (TMJ) pain in children is not common, but does present on occasions. Affected children complain of pain on eating, limited opening, locking or clicking. A careful history should be taken to enquire about other head, neck, joint or abdominal pain (which are common in these patients). In addition, questions should be asked about habits such as nail-biting, frequent gum-chewing, playing of wind instruments or a history of facial trauma, all of which may contribute to TMJ problems. Also, delicate enquiry needs to be made into the home, family and school situation to see if there could be underlying social or emotional problems. A full extraoral and intraoral examination, with in-depth assessment of asymmetry, muscle pain, jaw dynamics and occlusion, should follow. In the first instance, supportive advice and reassurance should be given about the following:

• soft diet
• analgesics (a non-steroidal anti-inflammatory preparation)
• application of a warm flannel or hot water bottle to the affected area

- avoidance of opening the mouth wide – for instance, during yawning
- no chewing gum
- cessation of nail- or pencil-chewing
- simple jaw-opening exercises.

If symptoms fail to improve, a soft occlusal splint may be provided. In some cases an orthodontic referral may be indicated if there is an underlying malocclusion.

Oral Lesions

At this point it should be stressed that children presenting with unusual oral lesions should receive urgent attention and appropriate referral for further investigation. In patients with oral lesions of concern, a more detailed history than usual may be indicated to include specific questions about general wellness, growth, fatigue, appetite loss, gastrointestinal symptoms and family medical history. Listed below are some of the clinical and radiographic features that may be seen in children with oral or underlying systemic disease. The limitation of this text means that differential diagnoses cannot be discussed, but references are given for more comprehensive reviews of paediatric oral medicine and pathology. In this text we can simply list some of the presenting signs or symptoms that warrant referral.

Clinical Features Justifying Specialist Referral
- pathologically mobile teeth, other than traumatised or abscessed teeth
- exceptionally premature eruption or exfoliation of teeth

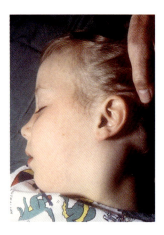

Fig 5-19 Six-year-old girl with Burkitt's lymphoma, presenting as a firm swelling in the left submandibular region.

- persistent or recurrent extra-oral swelling, other than due to an odonto-genic infection (Fig 5-19)
- submandibular lymphadenopathy, in the absence of an obvious cause such as recent viral infection, a dental abscess or ear infection
- paraesthesia
- intraoral swelling or lesion, other than periapical/periodontal abscesses
- generalised ulcerative or vesiculobullous lesions of the gingivae or mucosa
- abnormal gingival appearance, including diffuse swellings, haemorrhagic or granular presentations
- intraoral pigmented or vascular lesions
- spontaneous oral bleeding (in absence of a bleeding disorder or suspected acute herpetic gingivostomatitis).

Radiographic Features of Concern
- bony radiolucencies or opacities
- bony pathology associated with abnormal root resorption
- displacement of teeth by space-occupying lesions
- area of generalised bony rarefaction
- generalised or localised loss of alveolar bone support.

Recommended Reading

Andreasen JO, Andreasen FM. Textbook and Color Atlas of Traumatic Injuries to the Teeth. Copenhagen: Ed Munksgaard, 1994.

Cameron AC, Widmer RP. Handbook of Pediatric Dentistry. Edinburgh: Ed Mosby, 2003.

Hall RK. Pediatric Orofacial Medicine and Pathology. London: Chapman and Hall Medical, 1994.

Laskaris G. Color Atlas of Oral Diseases in Children and Adolescents. Stuttgart: Thieme, 2000.

Tsukiboshi M. Treatment planning for Traumatized Teeth. Chicago: Quintessence Publishing , 2000.

Welbury RR, Greeg T. Managing Dental Trauma in Practice. London: Quint-essence Publishing, 2005.

Chapter 6
Recall Strategy

Aim

This chapter will briefly discuss guidelines for planning recall schedules for children in general dental practice.

Outcome

On reading this section, the practitioner should be able to decide on an appropriate recall interval for an individual patient, taking into consideration social, medical and dental factors, including caries risk.

Introduction

Once the preventive and operative phase of a treatment plan has been completed, the young patient will, it is hoped, 'emerge' with a healthy dentition, knowledge of home-based prevention and a happy disposition towards dental treatment. Once things are stable, a recall appointment will need to be made. But how soon should the patient be seen again?

From a public health point of view, it is more efficient and economical to individualise and extend recall intervals for children, according to a clinical assessment of risk. As with treatment planning, one scheme does not fit all, so routinely prescribing six-month recall intervals for all children is neither efficient nor evidence-based.

The National Institute of Clinical Excellence (NICE) has produced detailed guidelines on dental recall intervals for both adults and children (www.nice.org.uk). It is recommended that the longest interval between recall for patients below 18 years is no more than 12 months. Conversely, a three-month recall is recommended for those assessed as high risk. The document also highlights the factors that should be considered when choosing recall intervals for individual patients. Interestingly, recent Scandinavian studies have recommended prolonging examination intervals to one-and-a-half to two years for some children at low risk. Indeed, extending recalls to 20 months did not appear to be detrimental to the dental health of many young patients.

This brief chapter simply aims to challenge practitioners to use their clinical judgement when deciding on recall intervals, rather than adopting the same protocol for all patients, regardless of clinical need. The following sections discuss the factors that might influence the timing of the recall examination, and include:

- caries risk
- medical status
- compliance
- stage of dental development
- specific dental conditions.

Caries Risk

An assessment of caries risk is fundamental to decision-making regarding recall intervals. Obviously, children who are categorised as at high risk of caries justify a shorter recall interval than those deemed to have low caries experience. Unless there are other clinical considerations (see below), the following recall schedule is suggested.

- low risk – recall nine to 12 months
- high risk – recall three to six months.

It is important to continually review caries risk at subsequent appointments and modify the recall interval accordingly. In particular, the clinician should monitor the activity of existing lesions and be alert to the development of new disease.

Compliance

Very young or anxious patients may benefit from shorter recall periods as part of a behaviour-shaping and acclimatisation strategy.

Medical Status

Patients with special needs or who are medically compromised, such as those with a bleeding disorder, congenital heart disorder or malignancy, obviously warrant a more frequent recall than those who are fit and well. Four- to six-monthly visits, with appropriate radiographic investigation, will ensure any caries is treated early, thus simplifying management and reducing the risk of serious complications. Furthermore, it may be necessary to adjust recall times to coincide with periods of wellness of the child, or other medical reviews.

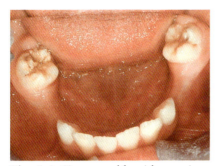

Fig 6-1 Six-year-old with previous extraction of carious primary molars and newly erupted hypoplastic first permanent molars: a good indication for early fissure-sealant placement.

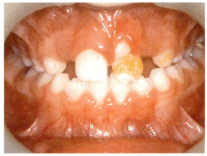

Fig 6-2 Eight-year-old with a history of trauma to primary incisors and resultant hypoplasia of upper left permanent central incisor: a restorative approach is needed.

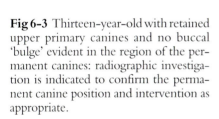

Fig 6-3 Thirteen-year-old with retained upper primary canines and no buccal 'bulge' evident in the region of the permanent canines: radiographic investigation is indicated to confirm the permanent canine position and intervention as appropriate.

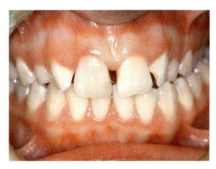

Dental Development

Recall appointments should not focus on caries assessment alone but should also provide an opportunity to monitor the development of the occlusion. There are some key stages of dental development when it would be prudent to recall the patient so that any interceptive treatment can be instigated if necessary. Children should be certainly be recalled more frequently around the following ages:

- Five to six years (Fig 6-1) to monitor the eruption and condition of the first permanent molars and to place fissure sealants for children at high risk of caries
- Eight to nine years (Fig 6-2) to monitor the eruption of the maxillary permanent incisors and palpate for maxillary canines
- Eleven to 12 years (Fig 6-3) to monitor the eruption of the maxillary permanent canines.

Once the occlusion is stable, following the eruption of the second permanent molars, it may be appropriate to consider a longer recall interval.

Specific Dental Conditions

Trauma
Another reason for a short recall interval (less than six months) may be past dental trauma experience. Trauma patients should be reviewed regularly to check for trauma-related sequelae, such as loss of vitality, inflammatory root resorption and eruption disturbances. Early detection of these complications and instigation of appropriate treatment is likely to improve overall prognosis.

Periodontal Disease
Obviously children with specific conditions, such as juvenile periodontitis, justify frequent recall and treatment as indicated clinically.

Dental Anomalies
Children with specific dental conditions, such hypodontia or enamel and dentine disorders, may require six-monthly recall - in particular, when extensive restorative treatment has been already undertaken and requires close review.

The Recall Appointment

The recall appointment should encompass more than just an examination; it should be used to:
- update social and medical histories
- carry out a thorough extra- and intraoral examination, including an assessment of oral hygiene and orthodontic status
- reassess caries risk
- take radiographs, if appropriate
- continue behaviour-shaping, if necessary
- reinforce dietary advice and oral hygiene instruction
- perform a preventive procedure, such as topical fluoride application, if indicated
- top up any deficient fissure sealants.

Summary

The frequency of recalls for children should be based on individual clinical need. Furthermore, the recall interval should be flexible and continually reassessed at subsequent attendances, depending on new clinical findings and risk assessment.

Recommended Reading

Lahti SM, Hausen HW, Widstrom E, Eerola A. Intervals for oral health examinations among Finnish children and adolescents: recommendations for the future. International Dental Journal 2001;51:57-61.

Wang NJ, Holst D. Individualizing recall intervals in child dental care. Community Dentistry and Oral Epidemiology 1995;23:1-7.

Wang NJ, Berger B, Ellingsen BH. Clinical judgement as a basis for choice of recall interval in child dental care? Community Dental Health 1998;15:252-255.

UK National Clinical Guidelines in Paediatric Dentistry. Continuing oral care: review and recall. International Journal of Paediatric Dentistry 1998;8:227-228.

Index

Toothache 103–105
Toothbrush 55, 56
Toothbrushing 55
Trauma 114
  and dental development 114, 115
  and treatment delay 115
  ankylosis 120
  facial fracture 120
  management 122–125
  orthodontic factors 117–119

prevention 49, 68, 69
review 132
root retention 116, 117
tooth colour changes 119
Treatment planning 15
  scenarios 17

V

Veneers 85, 86

Quintessentials for General Dental Practitioners Series

in 50 volumes

Editor-in-Chief: Professor Nairn H F Wilson

General Dentistry, Editor: Nairn Wilson

Implantology in General Dental Practice	available
Cultural and Religious Issues in Clinical Practice	Spring 2006
Dilemmas of Dental Erosion	Spring 2006
Managing Orofacial Pain in Practice	Autumn 2006
Denatl Bleaching	Autumn 2006

Oral Surgery and Oral Medicine, Editor: John G Meechan

Practical Dental Local Anaesthesia	available
Practical Oral Medicine	available
Practical Conscious Sedation	available
Practical Surgical Dentistry	Spring 2006

Imaging, Editor: Keith Horner

Interpreting Dental Radiographs	available
Panoramic Radiology	Spring 2006
Twenty-first Century Dental Imaging	Autumn 2006

Periodontology, Editor: Iain L C Chapple

Understanding Periodontal Diseases: Assessment and Diagnostic Procedures in Practice	available
Decision-Making for the Periodontal Team	available
Successful Periodontal Therapy – A Non-Surgical Approach	available
Periodontal Management of Children, Adolescents and Young Adults	available
Periodontal Medicine: A Window on the Body	Spring 2006

Endodontics, Editor: John M Whitworth

Rational Root Canal Treatment in Practice	available
Managing Endodontic Failure in Practice	available
Preventing Pulpal Injury in Practice	Autumn 2006

Quintessence Publishing Co. Ltd., London